D1446749

Nourishing the Soul of Pharmacy

Nourishing the Soul of Pharmacy

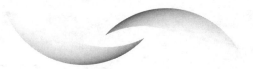

Stories of Reflection

Edited by

Thomas D. Zlatic, Ph.D.
William A. Zellmer, B.S. (Pharmacy), M.P.H.

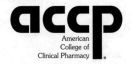

American College of Clinical Pharmacy
Lenexa, Kansas

Director of Professional Development: Nancy M. Perrin, M.A., CAE
Associate Director of Professional Development: Wafa Dahdal, Pharm.D., BCPS (AQ Cardiology)
Publications Project Manager: Janel Mosley
Graphic Designer/Desktop Publisher: Jen DeYoe, B.F.A.
Medical Editor: Kimma Sheldon, Ph.D., M.A.

For order information or questions, contact:
American College of Clinical Pharmacy
13000 West 87th Street Parkway, Suite 100
Lenexa, Kansas 66215
(913) 492-3311
(913) 492-0088 (Fax)
accp@accp.com

Disclaimer: The essays in this book are the personal reflections of pharmacy practitioners, composed from their own perspectives and rendered in their unique language and style. The views and opinions expressed in these essays are the authors' alone, and do not necessarily reflect those of the American College of Clinical Pharmacy or the editors. Names of individuals and details of patient cases have been changed to respect their privacy.

Copyright © 2011 by the American College of Clinical Pharmacy. No part of this publication may be reproduced, stored in a retrieval system, or transmitted, in any form or by any means, electronic or mechanical, including photocopy, without prior written permission of the American College of Clinical Pharmacy.

Printed in the United States of America
ISBN: 978-1-932658-83-5
Library of Congress Control Number: 2011938640

CONTENTS

CARE FROM THE OTHER SIDE OF THE COUNTER AND BEDSIDE:
PHARMACISTS AS PATIENTS AND CAREGIVERS

DIRE SITUATIONS: CARE AMID CATASTROPHE

CARE ACROSS CULTURES: MULTICULTURAL AWARENESS

TRUTH IN ACTION: ALTRUISM AND JUSTICE IN PHARMACEUTICAL CARE

GOOD INTENTIONS ARE NOT ENOUGH: LEARNING FROM OUR MISTAKES

EDUCATIONAL CARE: TEACHING, MENTORING, AND LEARNING

PHARMACY PROSPECTS: SHAPING THE FUTURE

RECOGNIZING LIMITATIONS

HUMANIZING THE PROFESSION

CELEBRATING PHARMACY

AFTERWORD

APPENDIX I

APPENDIX II

Preface

In January 2011, we put out a general call for papers in which authors reflect on clinical pharmacy.

Our goal was to stimulate activity in a type of reflective inquiry that would enhance empathy for patients and elicit deeper bonds between practitioners. This is part of a larger effort to humanize pharmacy practice as it continues to evolve in the direction of a patient-centered ethos.

Within weeks, dozens of inquiries arrived; a total of 140 essays were submitted, written by pharmacy clinicians, faculty, residents, and students. Selecting 69 for inclusion was difficult.

One reason is that we had a specific model of reflection in mind. Many submissions were excellent expository essays that covered important issues, but they were not "reflection" as we were defining the term. We also were not looking to produce a "feel-good" coffee-table book of warm and perhaps amusing anecdotes; though many selected essays are inspiring, others are troubling. And although some selected pieces are very well crafted, we were not requiring reflections to be literary masterpieces.

Instead, we were most interested in inquiry through narrative. "Reflection" in this volume refers to stories, particularly of patient encounters, that lead to complex insight and improved patient care.

To demonstrate that such reflections can be valuable at all stages of education and practice, we selected representative essays from senior professors and beginning faculty, pharmacy directors and new clinicians, preceptors and residents, Pharm.D. students and practitioners from industry and government. It is clear that all career levels, critical reflection on pharmacy situations can lead to greater patient empathy and the development of a professional culture that values patient-centered care.

Thus, the book is intended for a variety of audiences: practitioners, educators, and students and perhaps for patients, caregivers, and health care professionals seeking a better understanding of pharmacists and the roles they perform. For educators who might wish to adopt the volume as a supplementary textbook, an appendix for using reflection as a learning strategy is included.

We are grateful to all who submitted reflections, those that are printed in this book and those that may eventually appear in other publications. We are especially appreciative of faculty who encouraged and assisted students in the drafting of their reflections. And finally, we acknowledge with deep gratitude the tireless efforts of Janel Mosley, who cheerfully coordinated the collection and processing of so many submissions.

We envision that the success of our efforts will be assessed not upon the completion of this book, a product, but upon the initiation of a process. It is clear that there are many pharmacists who have stories to tell and want to tell them. We hope that this book might motivate ongoing efforts to develop habits of mind and practice that lead to empathic patient care.

Thomas D. Zlatic, Ph.D.
William A. Zellmer, B.S. (Pharmacy), M.P.H.

Introduction

Reflecting on the Mission of Pharmacy

Thomas D. Zlatic, Ph.D.

> Depth, value, relatedness, heart, and personal substance.
> People want and need pharmacists with those characteristics—
> pharmacists with soul. Let's dedicate ourselves to remaking this
> occupation of ours into a profession that gives people what they
> want and need.
>
> William A. Zellmer, *Searching for the Soul of Pharmacy*

In 1996, William Zellmer wrote insightfully that pharmacy was "an occupation on its way to becoming a profession" (354). For Zellmer, a crucial first step in that journey is an authentic professional commitment to patients.

I think another way of saying this is that what makes a health care professional is a patient. There are many definitions of "profession," but in its essence, a profession can be conceived as a unique type of relationship. What distinguishes a profession from an occupation is the differing relationships that pertain between providers and those they serve. Workers in an occupation have a mercantile relationship with customers; their primary responsibility is toward their employers or shareholders. Our "customers may always be right," as we assert with some cynicism, but our loyalty is toward those who pay our salaries. People in a profession have a covenantal or fiducial relationship with patients, clients, students, congregations. They do not have customers. Their primary obligation is a "faith" or "fiducial" relationship to the persons they serve (Zlatic, "Reaffirming the Human Nature of Professionalism"). In exchange for the patient's "gift of trust," the professional promises to work in the patient's best interest (American Pharmacists Association, Code of Ethics for Pharmacists). It is this special relationship that defines a profession. Again, it is the patient that makes the professional.

The transition from an occupation to a profession parallels pharmacy's transition from a product-oriented ethos to a patient-centered practice (Reich). Although the small-town community pharmacist or "doc" of the first half of the twentieth century often was personally involved in the lives of patients, pharmacy's emergence as a specialized product-oriented practice provided less incentive to encourage practitioners to reflect on their interactions with patients. Now, with pharmacy's expanded mission to provide pharmaceutical care and to assume responsibility for drug therapy outcomes, it is becoming apparent that at both the educational and practice levels, it is important for pharmacists to develop habits of mind that are wider and deeper in scope than clinical problem solving. To deal with patients who are more than chemicals, hormones, organs, or disease states, pharmacists need to be open to reflection on both clinical and human issues. For practitioners to care for and about patients, they need a supportive culture and a formational program that predispose them to respond not simply to drug problems or medical complaints but to patients in all of their human complexity.

For almost a century and a half, liberal education has been promoted in pharmacy education, sometimes with misguided motivations, such as trying to provide the pharmacist a finishing school–type cultural veneer to earn the respect of patients and facilitate interaction with other health care professionals (Zlatic, Chair Report). Offering humanities as distinct courses certainly can be effective in increasing interpersonal skills, broadening social and cultural awareness, and refining ethical decision-making. But to develop "value, depth, and heart"—to encourage practitioners to care for and care about patients—it is more important to integrate professional and liberal or humanistic education (Association of American Colleges and Universities; Shulman; Zlatic, "Liberalizing Professional Education"). Humanistic education is not merely additive but transformative. As a recent article on empathy development in medical education proposes, "Empathy training and the humanities should not be situated outside the hard core of medicine" (Pedersen). To develop pharmacists with "soul," the relevant insights and strategies of humanistic education must be integrated with professional education.

Literature, for instance, can be an important resource for pharmacy. Although literature for many is merely entertainment or escape, it can also be a means for reflecting on the complexities, possibilities, and problems within practice, whether the literature be fiction, poetry, film, or personal accounts and meditations. In medicine, there is a long tradition of physicians who are poets, essayists, and storytellers such as John Stone or Richard Selzer, and, more recently, Rachel Naomi Remen in works such as *My Grandfather's Blessings: Stories of Strength, Refuge, and Belonging*; the value of such reflections is manifested in medical journals, such as the "Piece of My Mind" column in JAMA, whose short pieces often explore humanistic values and ethics within professional settings.

Pharmacy has had fewer such champions. Of course, pharmacy education has a different curricular structure and philosophy, and the tightly packed curriculum leaves little time for reflection, but it is also true that until recently, the pharmacist's restricted relationship with a "patient" made such reflection less crucial. An empathic connection to patients entails values, ethics, and emotions—increasingly important components of practice that are not easily developed within didactic or clinical settings.

When trying to answer the questions, "What Is Empathy, and Can It Be Taught," Howard Spiro asserted that "Empathy can be strengthened best through stories" (845). It is through our stories that we can extend and deepen the empathy so crucial for professional practice.

So, a story.

About a dozen years ago, I accompanied Dr. Michael Maddux to the county health department to inquire about opportunities for pharmacy students in service learning.

The director of the program was very helpful, suggesting several opportunities for our students, and then she began to relate a few stories regarding the kinds of problems the agency typically encountered.

She told us that they recently had received a rash of unwarranted 911 calls. People were dialing for relatively trivial medical problems, or they needed a ride to the hospital for a nonemergency event. It was not just the expense of sending an ambulance and crew that was of concern; the vehicles speeding down the streets with sirens blaring were a safety risk for the attendants, other drivers, and pedestrians. Another potential problem was the unavailability of an EMT vehicle if a true emergency developed. "Your husband was having chest pains and is now unconscious? We will get an ambulance there as soon as one is available."

I knowingly shook my head, lamenting the irresponsibility and self-centeredness of people who abuse systems designed to protect them and the rest of us.

The director looked at me slyly and continued. Last week, a woman called 911 because the faucet in her kitchen sink was dripping. My resentment toward "those people" was rising and approached hostility when I heard the next part of the story: the woman's daughter lived one block away. Like most people, I believe I am an empathic person, but I was not able to muster much empathy for this woman with the dripping faucet who was wasting taxpayers' dollars, my dollars, when her daughter could have taken care of her problem in 5 minutes without any expense or threat to public safety.

Until I learned more. Sitting back in her chair, the director told us the caller was an older woman, living alone. But the elderly woman worried about for how long. She knew her next residence would be the "home." Her daughter had been trying to persuade her for some time that she needed help with daily living, but the woman had thus far successfully put her off. She knew what an inability to stop the faucet from dripping would mean if her daughter found out. Like many other people her age, for her the "home" was a death sentence. A loss of autonomy, unfamiliar surroundings, a disconnect from lifelong memories, forced associations with strangers. Her reply to the daughter's concern that, living alone, her mother might get hurt or burn down the house is a common one: "I'd rather burn up in my own kitchen tomorrow than live the rest of my life in an institution."

I realized then that for this woman, the dripping faucet was a true emergency, as much as if she had fallen and broken her hip. Each drip was an announcement that her life as she knew it was coming to an end. It was not irresponsibility or parsimoniousness that dialed 911. It was panic.

Of course, sanctioning 911 calls for dripping faucets is not the answer. And the health department was wise enough to come up with a solution: they instituted a nonemergency emergency number, a "912," that could help individuals with non–life-threatening problems without the expense and danger of speeding ambulances.

Although I could not condone the elderly woman's actions, I now could understand them. I originally could not be empathic toward her because I did not understand her situation. Empathy involves putting yourself in another's position. Instead, I forced her into my position. I judged her on assumptions and biases that I brought to her story. My limited background precluded empathy. I could not put myself in her place. I did not have the facts. I did not have the experience.

One reason it is difficult to teach empathy is that all of our students are empathic already. As no doubt we all are. At least I have never met a student or faculty member who has acknowledged being non-empathetic. But it is clear from the above reflection that empathy is more than an orientation. It is also a skill involving critical thinking, maturation, and a diminishment in ego- and sociocentricity. And it is a function of experience. In broadening our experience, we enhance our potential for empathy.

"Experience is the best teacher." True. But, as a former professor of mine, Walter J. Ong, often warned, it can also be the worst. You can die from it. And regardless of our age and backgrounds, our experience is always inadequate for understanding or for empathizing with all people in all situations. Thus, it is often safer and more practical to continue learning some things from the experiences of others. Our imaginative participation in the thoughts and lives of other people through stories is a pathway to empathy. This is the power and relevance of stories, of literature, for health care.

The sharing of stories, observations, and insights is also important for professionalization—for the development of practitioners who care both for and about patients.

> Effective for professional socialization are one's own stories—
> personal disclosures of faculty's and students' professional
> experiences, reflections, struggles, rewards, and joys. The
> commitment, passion, excitement, anxiety, pride, and satisfaction
> conveyed through stories are often more compelling than data,
> charts, textbooks, and reports.
>
> Thomas D. Zlatic, *Inculcating Professionalism*

Reflections are not expository essays or clinical reports: they acknowledge that human emotion is necessary for in-depth understanding. Reading and writing and telling stories do not only engage the mind; they activate the senses, emotions, and imagination as well. They get us involved in the narration through vivid, sensory descriptions that don't simply tell us what happened but also show us; they help us experience vicariously, imaginatively, situations outside our personal reality and elicit an emotional response. They convey not "content" but experience within the fullness of the human life world. These reflections not only spring from consciousness but also are rooted in unconsciousness. Thus, they invoke memories and touch us at depths we cannot enunciate. They challenge our perspectives. They allow us to enter the perspective of another person, to see the world through someone else's eyes. They allow us to put ourselves in someone else's place. I don't just know what you mean; I feel what you mean. I've been there.

Such reflection culminates in insight. Writing itself, like dialogue, is a method of discovery, the truth of which is proclaimed in maxims such as "how do I know what I think until I see what I say," and "we write not to be understood but to understand." Writing reflections helps us organize and analyze our experience: the process uncovers complexities that we had not noticed before. Ultimately, reflections are future-oriented: they help us identify changes that can help us become better professionals and persons.

This collection of reflections is an effort to advance the type of education and practice that is required for a profession. Ideally, the writing and reading of these reflections on the joys, sorrows, failures, injustices, and successes encountered in pharmacy practice can open up the complexity of the pharmacy profession and perhaps inspire pharmacists toward more ethical, altruistic, and character-driven practice.[1]

Reflection as a Way of Knowing

> By three methods we may learn wisdom: First, by reflection, which is noblest; second, by imitation, which is easiest; and third by experience, which is the bitterest.

> Attributed to Confucius

Meditation is an art. For centuries in the Western world, a three-step method of meditation was common to both religion and literature: (1) composition of place, (2) analysis, and (3) application or response (Martz).

The devout Christian meditating on the death of Jesus on the cross would be encouraged to put herself imaginatively at Calvary—to hear

---

1 The ACCP White Paper on "Development of Student Professionalism" is reprinted in Appendix II.

the crowd cursing and the groaning, the sound of nails pounded into bone; to feel the sun bearing down and the dust blown in the air; to smell blood and gall; and to see expressions of terror and anger. This was the composition of place. Then, the Christian would reflect on why Jesus died on the cross, on the Fall and redemption, on her own sinfulness and indifference for which the cross was an antidote—this was the analysis. And finally, the response: she would determine what she needed to do with her life to respond to the love that was hung on the cross.

In a more secular spirit, a poet such as William Cullen Bryant would seek in nature sources of inspiration. He would describe, for instance, the fringed gentian (a late-blooming flower of the autumn), reflect on the lesson of hope and persistence to be learned from the flower, and then resolve:

> I would that thus, when I shall see
> The hour of death draw near to me,
> Hope, blossoming within my heart,
> May look to heaven as I depart.

William Cullen Bryant, To a Fringed Gentian

These meditations were meant to involve the whole person. As understood at the time, the faculties of the mind were memory, understanding, and will. The three stages of meditation were meant to involve each: memory governed composition of place; understanding was related to analysis; and will guided the application or response.

Today, in our more practical and perhaps more prosaic era, meditation is less ingrained in our thinking. However, newer understandings of reflection are reasserting the importance of self-interrogation for personal and professional development. Following the early lead of John Dewey, several contemporary theorists have formulated models of reflection that inform reflective teaching, reflective practice, and reflective learning.[2] Advocates of reflective practice in professional education encour-

---

2 Classic texts are Dewey, Schön, and Freire; these are discussed by Lyons. Also see Moon, Bolton, and DiRanna et al. Some writers distinguish reflection from reflexivity: "Reflection is an in-depth consideration of events or situations outside of oneself. . . . Reflexivity is finding strategies to question our own attitudes, through processes, values, assumptions, prejudices, and habitual actions, to strive to understand our complex roles in relation to others (Bolton 13). See also Jasper.

age practitioners to embrace a variety of strategies of critical reflection, not only to enhance their competence but also to examine practice with respect to professional mission and ethical norms. Reflective writing or journaling is sometimes incorporated in these models.

Such theories provide a foundation for continuing professional development (CPD), a process of professional self-learning promoted in the professions as an alternative to continuing education (Council on Credentialing, Rouse, Austin). Continuing professional development is a structured, iterative process of reflection, planning, action, and evaluation used to develop a habit of "reflective practice" that can enhance knowledge, skills, and values needed to become a more successful practitioner.

Along these lines, Graham Gibbs in the Gibbs Reflective Cycle proposes six stages for reflection that lead to improvement: (1) Description (what happened); (2) Feelings (what were you thinking and feeling); (3) Evaluation (what was good and bad about the experience); (4) Analysis (what sense can you make of the experience); (5) Conclusion (what else could you have done); and (6) Action Plan (if it arose again, what would you do) (Gibbs 1988).

In the Gibbs model, one can see some similarity to the earlier meditation process: composition of place (description, feelings), analysis (evaluation, analysis, conclusion), and response (planning). For the somewhat different sense of reflective writing in this collection of narratives by pharmacists, we propose a compressed framework of four components that invoke memory, understanding, and will: account/description, response, analysis, and planning.

1. Account. Describe the situation/event in a detailed, concrete, vivid way.
2. Response. Give a realistic emotional reaction to the situation without becoming overly sentimental or "schmaltzy" (this response can be implied rather than stated).
3. Analysis. Extract insight on self and on deep or complex issues derived from the situation, skirting the obvious and superficial.
4. Planning. Decide what changes might be made to enhance professional practice.

Like CPD, this approach to reflection through narrative is both retrospective and prospective: review the past to improve in the future; certainly, the approaches are complementary. However, for such narrative inquiry, the emphasis is on involving the total person in recalling and responding to an event, analyzing it, and resolving to improve in some way because of it.[3] The more narrow focus of this reflection is on developing a more humanistic, patient-centered practice. Self-assessment comes in the form of a story. It entails the sharing of experience that engages the senses, the mind, the heart, and the will, with the goal being not only knowledge but also wisdom. This type of reflection also serves more of a communal function: it creates bonds. The telling and hearing of stories is part of professional socialization. The stories define and transmit the values, goals, and ideals that shape the profession, that constitute its soul.

Thus, "reflection" in this collection does not refer to purely analytic investigations of self and circumstances; nor does it refer to essays that abstractly and objectively discuss topics related to practice. Reflection is not the same as exposition (which is meant to inform) or persuasion (which is meant to convince). The purpose of reflection is not to teach or preach. Rather, reflection focuses on one's own experiences and what he or she learned from them. It is not a soapbox. The writer does not instruct the audience but shares a story—conveys not just facts but also experience.

We should not be formulaic in our approach to reflective writing. There is no recipe or blueprint for reflection, and working through each of the above four components methodically probably would not produce an excellent result. Experience cannot easily be squeezed into neat templates, and not all experience can be explained—sometimes it must simply be shared and endured. In this collection, we are promoting a more humanistic meditation on particular, individual, professional experiences that help us better understand and embrace our professional roles and commitments.

To better understand the components of this type of reflection, we can analyze one of the essays contained in this book that provides a clear example of observation, emotional response, analysis, and planning.

Dr. Keri Sims in *"¿Como Se Dice . . . ?"* narrates her experience serving residents of a Guatemalan garbage dump (see p. 151). However, rather than taking a chronological approach and immediately narrating her story, Sims begins by announcing the insight she derived from her experience in Guatemala. What she is writing is not simply a travelogue

---

3 For arguments regarding narrative as a way of knowing, see Bruner; Lyons and Kubler LaBoskey.

but a record of her growth in interpersonal communication skills. That insight is what gives direction to the reflection. It determines what gets said and what does not get said, and it determines how the reflection is structured. It is clear this reflection will be analytic and introspective.

Account

Sims invokes memory to provide a "composition of place." That is, she gives a vivid, sensory description of her visit. She does not simply tell us about the place but also tries to get us to experience it through multisensory imagery:

> As we descended into the dump, the hills of garbage became mountains, and the air became more and more pungent and rancid. It was apparent that I would not be able to hold my breath for an hour, but I did tend to keep my mouth closed, fearing that I might taste the foulness of the air. We watched as men, women, and children left their stake in the garbage and raced to get in line for the little red pickup that brought lunch. . . . Vultures circled overhead. Packs of scrawny, grungy dogs and wild pigs scavenged through the garbage right beside the workers.

After probably 30 or more years, I still vividly recall a full-page magazine advertisement for a children's relief fund with a full-face picture of a young girl's face looking solemnly at the camera, under a caption that said something like, "You can save Emilia Cortez for $18 a month, or you can turn the page." We can get inured to reports of thousands of children suffering in poverty, but if we see a picture of one 5-year-old emaciated little girl, we are more likely to be moved to action, exemplifying the observation often attributed (erroneously) to Stalin: "The death of one man is a tragedy, the death of millions is a statistic." Sims does not talk about statistics; she shows us an ongoing tragedy.

Emotional response

Sims is not a passive, objective observer, as scientists and clinicians are sometimes trained to be. Embedded in her descriptive account is emotional response. She acknowledges her insecurity, discomfort, and perplexity. She identifies her fear of rejection that prevents her from opening herself up to the people she so much wants to help. But her response is not maudlin: she does not distort or oversimplify for the sake of vapid sentimentality. This is not a contrived tear-jerker movie that is "so good—I cried all the way through it."

Analysis

Sims does not simply look but sees. She analyzes. She can put herself in the place of the people inhabiting the garbage dump, imagining how humiliating it might be for them to be put on display like zoo animals for foreign visitors. She further recognizes that well-meaning volunteers can unwittingly be insulting or demeaning. Her empathy allows her to notice how we can become paralyzed by such awareness, how we can be unable to act for fear of failure or embarrassment. She is forced to recognize the irony: our efforts not to be offensive can cause us to be offensive.

She also learns about herself. She recognizes the need to enhance nonverbal communication. She then can extend to her practice the insight that the little girl from Guatemala taught:

> This interaction with the young girl helped me realize that so many of my patients "speak a different language." Granted, they speak English, but as inpatients on a Veterans Affairs Medical Center floor, they often speak a different dialect. Each patient's "dialect" is formed by his or her own personal experiences, struggles, desires, fears, and background. One's "dialect" may be influenced by having been in combat, another's by being homeless, and still another's by struggling with alcoholism or coping with multiple chronic diseases. I will never be able to fully understand every patient's dialect.

Planning

Reflection can be transformative. Insight leads to action. In this case, the outcome is better patient care:

That doesn't mean that I can't try to communicate with them. I can get over myself, venture into my uncomfortable zone and utilize the universal language of nonverbal communication. I have the opportunity to actually show that I care by sitting beside them, holding a hand or patting a knee. In doing so, I can break down some barriers that exist in our verbal communication as well.

Again, it is not necessary that every reflection programmatically include all four components of description, response, analysis, and planning. There is no formula for insight. What is needed is a willingness to openly, honestly, and critically explore and share one's ideas, actions, and values.

This storytelling approach is not meant to replace the cool detachment of reflective inquiry. Without critical awareness, stories of self-reflection can promote self-deception. Other modes of reflective thinking and practice can and should be employed to enhance personal and professional growth. The story is not a conclusion but an invitation to probe further, to reevaluate actions and belief systems, to question social and political structures, to identify and test assumptions, to systematically investigate issues further, to value open-mindedness and intellectual honesty, to monitor follow-through, and to assess progress.

Some types of knowing require distance or "distanciation"; others require immersion. Knowing and knowing about are complimentary but different. Both are necessary to avoid sterile rationalism and trite sentimentality. Reflective narrative can serve as a vehicle for humanizing and thus enhancing patient care and perhaps advancing the altruistic principles of servant leadership that are embedded in some deeper understandings of professionalism. Such reflections can nourish the "soul" of pharmacy.

This Collection

The response to our call for reflections was heartening—heartening not simply for wary editors concerned about the viability of such a project, but heartening also because of what it says about the profession. The fact that there were enough submissions to fill a couple of volumes signals an untapped interest of people who have stories to tell and who want to tell them—pharmacy students, residents, clinicians, faculty, practitioners. We are impressed by the range of the reflections and, particularly, the depth and commitment they demonstrate. Reading and responding to so many thought-provoking stories is an experience that is itself worthy of reflection.

Many pharmacists have experienced the joy of establishing human connections in professional settings, admiration for the dignity and courage of those suffering, and the pain of personal loss when the relationship ended, too often at death (Puet, Powell, Lemay, K. Smith, Burghardt, Morello). As Dinolfo says, "If you want to distill your temperament, your strengths, your weaknesses—the little vagaries that make you, you—into some pure, lit-from-within essence, try fighting a life-threatening illness. My God, the capacity for joy, the sense of appreciation, the humor, the courage—I had never seen anything like it."

If a goal of reflection is empathy, perhaps it is most deeply realized when the providers become the patient or caregiver—when they move to the other side of the counter or bedside. A reflection that begins, "A pharmacist killed my grandmother," promises hard-won insight that will last a lifetime (McClendon). Caring for a terminal patient who has been a longtime family friend (Belavic), watching a grandmother undergo medical mishaps (K. Smith), taking care of a mother with chronic heart and lung problems (Goldwater), or suffering oneself from a chronic illness (Fitz) teaches lessons of empathy, care, and commitment that cannot be learned from textbooks and lectures. On a more everyday level, when a new mother coming home from the hospital stops at a pharmacy and is told by the pharmacist that he is too busy to retrieve a bottle of ibuprofen, she wonders about how often she failed to serve her patients to the best of her ability because, she says, "I had not yet experienced the birth of my first child and all the love, worries, and special moments that came into my life when she did" (Ellis).

Reflection is heightened by times of stress, so it is not surprising that many submissions deal with catastrophic situations such as natural disasters (Harger, Minor, Wicker), war (Yam, Sucher), medical missions (Arif, Sims), and dire medical situations (Taylor). Some of these experiences can be life-changing. Wietholter writes of a medical trip to South Africa:

As a student at the University of Pittsburgh, I was the kid that sat at the back of the classroom: the kid that did crossword puzzles and Sudoku puzzles instead of fully immersing myself in lectures; the kid that occasionally nodded off during class, dreaming of the big payday upon completion of pharmacy school. I was not going to teach. . . . And then, in a brief 2-week period on the other side of the world, everything changed.

However, with attention, one can find insight and commitment in the more mundane and commonplace (Taylor); it is often the "little things" that count, as Pon learns in Haiti. What one local schoolteacher was most appreciative of were eyedrops for a chronic eye irritation:

> It was the simplest of things—artificial tears—nothing heroic, nothing life-saving, nothing to write home about. And yet, it was the most rewarding experience of my trip. For a moment, I was able to view the work that we were trying to do in that little village from the perspective of a villager, rather than from my own lofty, idealistic perspective. Maybe it really was the little things in life that made a difference.

The reflections demonstrate that pharmacy services can be given in a wide variety of settings and practices, including geriatrics (Estus, Portokalis), oncology (Dinolfo), trauma ICU (Belavic), community pharmacy (Lemay), and even a courtroom (Artymowicz). Although acknowledging, with perhaps a bit of ironic understatement, that "The federal government is not the first place people turn when they lose a loved one due to a medication error," Davison nonetheless convincingly portrays how a pharmacist at an FDA call center can be "a source of kindness, understanding, and empathy to callers who have experienced an adverse event." Sometimes, care can be masked but still be expressed by humor, even wry or self-protective "gallows" humor (Lynch; Butler and Kennedy).

Insights on the impact of culture on health care are registered by several authors: McLaughlin-Middlekauff on Alaska; Vongspanich on Africa; Torres and Rodríguez on Puerto Rico; Held on Palestine. Draeger reflects on the unique medical problems of an expanding subculture: the homeless. Frequently, these encounters dramatize social injustice (Harger). Jonkman pricks our social consciences in her moving account of an African woman who died because she had "no guardian," a metonymy for the lack of resources and injustice in the poverty-stricken nation: "she died because she was a woman, because she was African, and because she was poor. She had no voice, no one to speak up for her, no one to fight her battles."

A lingering sense of personal guilt, whether deserved or not, propels some reflections. Long lasting are memories of personal mistakes—failures in knowledge, skills, courage, or confidence—that led to negative patient outcomes (Pon as a "Wimpy Pharmacist"; Yocum and Haines; Huggins). But those memories also lead to deep and firm resolutions to become more determined and committed patient providers and advocates.

Some reflections contemplate the direction of pharmacy and its expanding roles (Shealy). Important in this expansion are allies, including health care professionals (Milavetz, Kelley) and patient champions (Padilla). Pharmacists must also recognize their own potential to "sell" pharmacy to patients and health care providers (Coppenrath). Observing that "there are no pharmacists on *Star Trek*," Zabriskie hooks an alternative future for pharmacy to patients' need and desire for the "personal interventions of a pharmacist," though apparently, it is a problem trying to convince all pharmacy students that this is the case (Brewer and Denvir). In face of expanding opportunities, it is important to find a balance in one's personal and professional life (Murphy, Ogden, Alexander). Some reflections (Ruch, Ponte, Henneberry on "Beauty in Change") are simply lyrical and celebratory about the profession.

Education is a source of reflection for students, residents, and faculty. Topics include the need to be open to new teaching strategies (Sommi, Gal) and the importance of mentors who model what pharmacy can be (Kabat, Chuk, Bystrack). Pharmacy educators have fiducial obligations not only to patients but also to students; Pesaturo reflects on the challenge of determining what it means to act in the best interest of the student who is not performing. Lindblad as a preceptor recognizes that with a change in her perspective, students can be helpful colleagues rather than a drain on one's time. Flannery's discovery of the importance of patient education changes her approach to patient care. Other contributors testify to the need for reflective (Kristeller) and right-brain thinking (Knoderer) in pharmacy education.

Some experiences provide further evidence that often, good intentions are not enough. Koenig astutely recognizes that her indignation and anger regarding her students' discomfort and ridicule toward homeless patients should be replaced by strategic mentoring. Allen, "humbled in Haiti," realizes that her quest for a good feeling, her desire to be a hero, got in the way of helping.

Sometimes most compelling—and disturbing—are reflections that raise questions rather than answer them. Then, reflection does not lead to resolution but to recognition of complexity and limitations. Behind textbook celebrations and admonitions regarding empathy lie painful human realities, as Wilken discovers in a smoking cessation clinic in a rough side of Chicago:

> I once had a sociology professor in college who said people with psychiatric illnesses were not really the ill people. The people that can watch all of the madness in the world and still have a smile on their faces were really the sick people. Now I understand. Doctors, priests, social workers, and now pharmacists are in positions where they are asked to really listen to each person. It is painful and difficult to hear the truth, so we become numb. This numbness is not intentional or vicious; it is a means of survival. My smile has to be indifferent. Should I stop smiling? I believe the patients need some form of hope. Should I change jobs?

And in "Faith?," Janning, faced with a patient's refusal of medical treatment on the basis of religious principles, can't explain but ponders nonetheless what compels one to die for one's faith:

> I have no doubt that many, perhaps most, suicide bombers are mentally ill individuals, many of whom are victimized by political extremists to conduct heinous acts in the name of their God. I do not at all believe that any true religion, as I understand the concept, advocates retribution against anyone by means of random mass murder. But I absolutely believe that, for a few, there exists a depth of faith that is literally worth dying for. I've seen it.

Henneberry's brief encounter with a dying VA patient who insists, against his doctor's advice, on being released to the care and home cooking of his beloved wife elicits not only understanding but also wisdom: "And so it was that a 15-minute experience with a patient changed my perspective on health care. I could no longer think of patients as we had in school, on paper, fitting neatly into therapy regimens we set, also on paper. Patients, I realized, are each their own story. They come to us at different chapters in their stories."

Such reflections can be cathartic, as writing can give some order to the experience. Sharing an experience also can lead to a type of emotional understanding that is somehow comforting. Perhaps at some level, all of these stories are a recognition that as human beings, we are fallible, limited, finite, incomplete, and contingent. Not logic nor knowledge nor good intentions can solve all our problems, can save us. Neither can our stories. But through our stories we can establish bonds, and it is this connection of one individual to another that can underpin a profession.

Works Cited

American Pharmacists Association. Code of Ethics for Pharmacists. Washington, DC: American Pharmacists Association, 1994.

Association of American Colleges and Universities. Taking Responsibility for the Quality of the Baccalaureate Degree. A Report from the Greater Expectations Project on Accreditation and Assessment. Washington, DC: Association of American Colleges and Universities, 2004.

Austin Z. Continuing professional development and lifelong learning. In: Zlatic TD, ed. Clinical Faculty Survival Guide. Lenexa, KS: American College of Clinical Pharmacy, 2010:chap 21.

Bolton G. Reflective Practice: Writing and Professional Development. Los Angeles: Sage, 2010.

Bruner J. Actual Minds, Possible Worlds. Cambridge, MA: Harvard University Press, 1986.

The Council on Credentialing in Pharmacy. Continuing Professional Development in Pharmacy. Washington, DC: The Council on Credentialing in Pharmacy, April 2004.

Dewey J. How We Think: A Restatement of the Relation of Reflective Thinking to the Educative Process. Boston: D.C. Heath and Company, 1910.

DiRanna K, Osmundson E, Topps J, Barakos L, Gearhart M, Cerwin K, Carnahan D, Strang C. Assessment-Centered Teaching: A Reflective Practice. Thousand Oaks, CA: Corwin Press, 2008.

Freire P. Pedagogy of the Oppressed. Bergman Ramos M, trans. New York: Seabury Press, 1970.

Gibbs G. Learning by Doing: A Guide to Teaching and Learning Methods. Further Education Unit. Oxford: Oxford Polytechnic, 1988.

Jasper M. Beginning Reflective Practice: Foundations in Nursing and Health Care. Cheltenham, UK: Nelson Thomas, 2003.

Lyons N. Handbook of Reflection and Reflective Inquiry: Mapping a Way of Knowing for Professional Reflective Inquiry. New York: Springer, 2009.

Lyons N, Kubler LaBoskey V, eds. Narrative Inquiry in Practice: Advancing the Knowledge of Teaching. New York: Teachers College Press, 2002.

Martz L. The Poetry of Meditation: A Study in English Religious Literature of the Seventeenth Century. New Haven: Yale University Press, 1962.

Moon JA. A Handbook of Reflective and Experiential Learning. London: RoutledgeFalmer, 2004.

Pedersen R. Empathy development in medical education—a critical review. Med Teach 2010;32:593–600.

Reich WT. What "care" can mean for pharmaceutical ethics. In: Haddad AM, Buerki RA, eds. Ethical Dimensions of Pharmaceutical Care. Binghamton, NY: Pharmaceutical Products Press, 1996:1–17.

Remen RN. My Grandfather's Blessings: Stories of Strength, Refuge, and Belonging. New York: Riverhead Books, 2000.

Roth MT, Zlatic TD. Development of student professionalism. White Paper, American College of Clinical Pharmacy. Pharmacotherapy 2009;29(6):749–56.

Rouse M. Continuing professional development in pharmacy. Am J Pharm Educ 2004;44:517–20.

Schön D. The Reflective Practitioner: How Professionals Think in Action. New York: Basic Books, 1983.

Selzer R. The Doctor Stories. New York: Picador, 1998.

Shulman LS. Professing the liberal arts. In: Orrill R, ed. Education and Democracy: Re-imaging Liberal Learning in America. New York: The College Board, 1997.

Spiro H. What is empathy and can it be taught? Ann Intern Med 1992;116:843–6.

Stone J. In the Country of Hearts: Journeys in the Art of Medicine. Baton Rouge: Louisiana State University Press, 1996.

Zellmer WA. Searching for the soul of pharmacy. Am J Health Syst Pharm 1996;53:1911–6.

Zlatic TD. Integrating education: chair report for the Academic Affairs Committee. Am J Pharm Educ 2000;64(winter suppl):8S–15S.

Zlatic TD. Liberalizing professional education: integrating general and professional ability outcomes. J Pharm Pract 2000;13:365–72.

Zlatic TD. Inculcating professionalism. In: Zlatic TD, ed. Clinical Faculty Survival Guide. Lenexa, KS: ACCP, 2010:193–207.

Zlatic TD. Reaffirming the human nature of professionalism. In: Zlatic TD, ed. Clinical Faculty Survival Guide. Lenexa, KS: ACCP, 2010:3–20.

Nourishing the Soul of Pharmacy

The Human Condition

The Joy and Pain of Patient Interaction

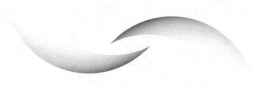

*Suffering and joy teach us, if we allow them,
how to make the leap of empathy, which
transports us into the soul and heart of
another person.*

Fritz William

*Yet, taught by time, my heart has learned
to glow for other's good, and melt at
other's woe.*

Homer

Can I Get a Witness?

Melissa Dinolfo, Pharm.D., BCOP
Clinician/Researcher

Eight years ago, I was a full-time mom, having served 11 years of hard time taking care of our two kids, clinging desperately to my dwindling brainpower along with my sanity.

Here's the thing about parenthood. When you are used to actually achieving something tangible with your days, and having some vague idea of how you have performed, and even having some discretionary cash to buy those shoes you have had your eye on at Nordstrom, parenting is a tough transition. No one stops you in the produce section of Ralph's to compliment you on your masterful handling of your 3-year-old son's tantrum—which has rendered him speechless, hiccupping in grief over your failure to provide him with a donut, with a torrent of snot streaming down his face. No one notices, or cares, that your peanut butter and jelly sandwiches have the perfect amount of each ingredient and that the crusts are precisely cut to your kindergartner's rigorous standards. And, when you are expected to be within a fraction of a percentage of precision on any drug preparation, how in the world do you navigate a recipe that includes the palpitation-inducing phrase "season to taste"?

One more thing about parenthood—perhaps the most important thing of all. Children, in their random, erratic, terrible glory, defy the parent to create a construct that simultaneously allows creative exploration while ensuring viability. Because my entire pharmacy career was about being a gatekeeper and keeping others safe, my children experienced a level of scrutiny that would have earned me a resounding "exceeds expectations" on my annual parental evaluation, had such a tool existed. But what about my poor kids? For the first 10 years or so, my oversight was a blessing, but as time spooled forward and they needed to actually experience a few rough patches and make their own mistakes, my loving, well-intentioned efforts began to chafe. However, as much as I tried, I lacked the discipline, or perhaps the perspective, to clear-cut the canopy and give them light to bloom, particularly as there was nothing of substance to occupy the void that such a transition would create. I needed something more.

So, with my sweet husband's blessing and at the august age of 47, I reentered the workforce. In my naïveté (which, unfortunately, I possess in abundance), I decided to accept a position as an "investigational drug pharmacist" for an oncology practice conducting clinical trials in patients with cancer, operating under the assumption that because the compounds were investigational, and therefore not well known, my own lack of recent work experience would not be as evident.

Disaster. The previous "investigational drug pharmacist" had resigned several months earlier (having held the position for only a few months, a red flag of which I was blissfully unaware), so there was no one to train me…literally. Each drug came with a multipage guide describing how it was manufactured, and basically, I was pointed in the direction of the hood and told to get to it.

Now, I'm not modest. I know I have gifts, and I am happy to use them. Unfortunately, though, in my years as a "clinical" pharmacist, mingling among patients, functioning as part of a multidisciplinary team, I had let what little IV skills I possessed lapse. To find myself in a chemo hood handling strange substances with all sorts of quirks and idiosyncrasies was a nightmare of epic proportions—what had I been thinking?

The third day—this is no lie—I had to manufacture a liposomal formulation of a drug that required, among other things, 2 hours tethered to a laboratory platform shaker, agitating at a ridiculously rapid rate, all in an effort to coax the reluctant components into some sort of cloudy coherence. The protocol had specified a certain model of shaker, but the practice I worked for, in an attempt to limit costs, had elected not to use it, instead adapting one they had on hand. As the fit was not quite right, I decided to use a foam baffle on the shaker to keep the bottles from breaking. I painstakingly cut a foam block with holes for my four little 100-mg bottles, proudly loaded them, and set the timer. In my zeal, I did not foresee that my jerry-rigged cushioning system would also function to insulate the vials and create enough friction that they would emerge, 2 hours later…boiling. Literally, there was steam condensing on the walls of all four bottles.

Here's another thing about phase I investigational drugs. Depending on the degree of OCD possessed by the sponsor, you could have a variety of stability data to evaluate, but sometimes, there might only be the recommendation that the drug was good at 8°C, with the moon in Virgo, on a Tuesday. To my endless humiliation, this sponsor had not had the foresight to boil the drug to see if it held up, and since I had no data, and making the drug again would take another 4 hours, I had to tell the clinic to cancel the treatment. This was my third day.

Fast-forward 4 weeks. I have lost 5 pounds and have diarrhea the night before I have to mix anything new. The treatment nurses are dropping into the prep area and saying things like "Aren't you done yet?", which is a real confidence-booster, believe me. I cry on the shoulder of a neighbor, a psychologist, and she says in a syrupy, patronizing way, "But Melissa, it can't be that important, can it?" Whereupon I reply, with some heat, "Eileen, the things I make with my two hands go directly into the bodies of dying people." There is a pregnant pause, and then she says only "Oh."

At about that time, I started venturing outside my little hood to the treatment area. It was there that I found something unexpected, something miraculous, and something that sealed my fate—hook, line, and sinker—and has brought me here today.

I found the patients.

If you want to distill your temperament, your strengths, your weaknesses—the little vagaries that make you, you—into some pure, lit-from-within essence, try fighting a life-threatening illness. My God, the capacity for joy, the sense of appreciation, the humor, the courage—I had never seen anything like it. Add to that the loving dread, anxiety, and hope evinced by the family; the mutual refusal to capitulate to terror; the tender, funny exchanges while walking together to the bathroom, pushing the IV pole…day by day, I saw everything noble, remarkable, and beautiful that is, or can be, life. It resides in the eyes of those who know their time is limited, and it gives them a vibrancy, intensity, and vulnerability that will take your breath away.

As I write this, I think of Hilary, who had developed breast cancer at age 42 while 5 months pregnant with her third child. The obstetrician to whom Hilary had reported her breast lump had dismissed it as a clogged milk duct and continued to do so even as it doubled in size, until by the time her little son was born, it comprised her entire left breast. She found herself in our clinic when her baby was barely 2 weeks old, being told that she had stage IV breast cancer with massive, crippling metastasis to her bones. I, as anyone would be, was so horrified by these developments that I always made a point to give her extra time for questions—or just to help her process the latest news from her doctor. One day, I was hesitating, trying to choose a word that wouldn't overly emphasize how dire things were, when she looked me straight in the eye and said, "Tell me everything, no matter how bad. It will help me fight harder."

To this day, I can't adequately describe the impact of her words on me. In that split second, I partnered with her in an unspoken promise that I would fight as long, and as hard, as she could. That I would try to be authentic in my relationship with her so that she could have a springboard to bounce things off of that might be too hard for her husband and family to hear. And, in so doing, I learned that people struggling with terrible illnesses need a companion, a safe place, a keeper of confidences. This is the toughest stuff of life, and it awaits all of us. Yet while we rail against it, each of us deserves a witness.

So, I mastered my job. In fact, I got good enough to actually go out into the clinic and talk to patients and work with them to help them relieve their suffering, stay strong and, sometimes, to let go. I learned that although we can't fix everybody, we can give our patients the dignity, respect, and honesty of seeing them through, of traveling with them, of telling them—when our efforts have failed—that we are sorry, and of saying goodbye. I am blessed beyond measure to be part of it. It has lent my life a texture, richness, and sense of perspective and simplicity that put my own disappointments in order. It has helped me grow as a parent, a wife, and a friend. It has humbled me and taught me to share my own doubts, sorrows, and misgivings. And, as hard as it is, as much as I have cried for all of those wonderful people who have allowed me to accompany them on their final journey, I have only the deepest, and most tender, gratitude.

An Untouched Phone Number

Brandi Puet, Pharm.D.
Clinician

I was sitting on the floor 7 months pregnant, surrounded by piles of small pink heaps of clothing, diapers, and blankets. I was exhausted from the 6-hour drive I had just completed. My remaining energy was from excitement over my loot and determination to complete the task at hand. I had spent the past weekend in my hometown to attend a baby shower in my honor. It was a wonderful shower full of family and friends, an immense array of salty foods (to appease a woman currently appalled by sweets), gifts with pale pink wrapping and bows, and cakes made of diapers and pacifiers. Now I was completing the dreaded task of filling out thank you cards. To make sure I conveyed my deepest gratitude, I was painstakingly reviewing every thank you card at least twice and adding a personal touch to each and every card. "Dear Aunt Judy, Thank you so much for the three outfits, bibs, and socks. I especially loved the pants with the cat on the back of them. Charleigh will look so cute in them. It was so great to see you at the shower. Thank you for sharing in our excitement over the baby. Thank you again. Love, Brandi." As I went to seal the envelope, I realized Aunt Judy also included a package of pacifiers with her gift. I picked up a new thank you card and rewrote: "Dear Aunt Judy, Thank you so much for the three outfits, bibs, socks, and pacifiers...." This compulsive tendency and attention to detail are partly due to my personality, the same personality traits that attract many pharmacists to enter the profession and make them so good at their jobs. I also blame the pregnancy hormones and the panic driving me to get everything done before the life-changing event took place. Either way, the thank you cards had to be perfect and completed that day before a single baby item could be put away (after being thoroughly washed, of course). It was during this moment that I realized there was someone missing at my shower. Someone I had not spoken to in quite some time. I pushed the thought to the back of my mind since I was a pregnant woman on a mission to finish the task at hand. The next day, I decided to make the phone call.

I had sent Ms. Betty a card 9 months earlier and never heard back from her. This was not typical of her. I usually receive a four-page letter in response, with hard-to-read, shaky handwriting. I had put off this call for months. Ms. Betty was in her 80s and in failing health. I wasn't sure if I really wanted to know how she was. My fears were confirmed when I called. The operator's monotone voice announced, "This number has been disconnected." I broke out in tears, convinced she had passed away and hurt that her family had never called me.

It took several days to build up the nerve to contact her family. To my relief, Ms. Betty had just moved to live closer to one of her daughters. Unfortunately, Ms. Betty's dementia had significantly worsened. According to her daughter-in-law, she had a strong memory of things long ago but very little memory of the past few years. I was certain this meant she had no recollection of me. I spoke awhile with her daughter-in-law, wrote down Ms. Betty's new number, and gave her family my new contact information to reach me if anything ever happened to her.

Ms. Betty was my "patient" when I was a pharmacy student. I was assigned to visit her for 2 hours once a week as part of our "patient practice experience." I fell in love with her the first time I met her and immediately adopted her as my grandmother away from home. She was a short, cute woman with fluffy gray hair that had been curled and sprayed stiff. Her sparkling green eyes and bright smile hid a life of hardship and losses. She had spent more than 20 years in an abusive marriage, a marriage that she had abandoned once her children were grown. Her first child was stillborn, and she was told during her grief by an uncompassionate physician, "You better never try to have children again!" She recalled resisting the urge to show up on his doorstep years later with her four beautiful, healthy children. Her stories were told with such vivid detail that I was almost convinced I had lived through them, also.

Her heart and mind were constantly with her family, and she spent many hours worrying and praying over them. I felt that I personally knew them all from hearing about them repeatedly. Never have I seen anyone love and care for their family as much as she did. Her love was not unrewarded. I could tell through the way her children fussed over her, spoke to her, and looked at her lovingly that they also loved and cherished her. I could tell you each and every name of her children and grandchildren and details about them.... "Richard is her oldest and the only male child. He just retired from the army and has a daughter named Amy and son, Brad. Amy is married to her second husband, and they have two wonderful boys, Sam and David. David has a heart condition. Brad is currently manager at the local grocery store and is engaged. The whole family is not sure about his new fiancé...." One day when she called after me as I was leaving, I realized she worried over me, also. "Brandi!" I looked back and said, "Yes ma'am?" "You know how you call me before you come to visit me every time?" (This was a necessity to ensure she was at home; she lived 30 minutes away and had a better social life than I did.) "Yes ma'am." "Do you mind calling me when you get home, so I know that you make it back safely?" I did just that and continued to do so after each visit.

My 2-hour visits usually turned into 4-hour visits. She made dinner for me on most visits and an occasional pound cake. She always commented on how she "messed up" the biscuits or did not add enough seasoning to the beans, but her meals were perfect; what graduate student would ever complain about a home-cooked meal!

Ms. Betty also had a fascinating health history. She was allergic to almost every antibiotic made and to several other medications. She had a history of anaphylaxis to penicillin and hives for the other medications on her allergy list. She also saw multiple doctors who did not always keep track of what her other doctors were doing. About the only skill I had at the time was the ability to take a blood pressure, and I had limited drug knowledge. Armed with my short white coat and love for her, I put all I could into researching her disease states, keeping track of her medications, and, of course, taking her blood pressure. My efforts paid off. I was able to intervene on a couple of near misses. She was given a first-generation cephalosporin on one occasion, for which I called her physician due to her previous near-fatal reaction to penicillin. She also called me one day to notify me that she had hives, and I discovered at the time that she had been given Levaquin despite a history of hives to Cipro. I also spent hours filling out forms for her to receive free medications due to her low income. Not to mention the painful experience of her family and me trying to figure out a Medicare Part D plan for her.

Ms. Betty thought I was the best "little pharmacist" she had ever seen. I grew in confidence seeing that my efforts and knowledge were benefiting someone else. I became passionate for my profession, seeing how much faith and trust she had in me. I could not imagine making it through my pharmacy school years without her words of encouragement and praise.

It was a bittersweet day when I left my college town to go on rotations, knowing that I would be too busy and too far away to return to my college town. I took great efforts to influence who my predecessor would be. I did not trust Ms. Betty with just any pharmacy student. I talked to Ms. Betty several times the following year. She ended up having three students that came to see her on a rotating schedule. She was sure to tell me that none of them was as good as me. It humbled me to hear the way she referred to her students. It was truly that she saw them as "her students." I realized that she was teaching them just like she taught me.

I have now been out of school for 4 years and have a wonderful husband and sweet baby girl. Ms. Betty would love to have known all of this. Ms. Betty's number is still tucked away in my desk drawer untouched.

A Pharmacist's Gift

Virginia A. Lemay, Pharm.D., CDOE
Educator/Community Pharmacist

"Cystic fibrosis is a cruel disease." These were the words my patient spoke who had just lost her 16-year-old daughter to the complications of cystic fibrosis.

Having practiced in a community pharmacy since high school, I have interacted with thousands of patients. Through the years, I have developed a profound patience and a deep respect for all people and their ailments. I have delivered medication to those who were unable to leave their homes. I have traveled to my patients' homes to replace their safety caps with non-safety caps, because their hands were too weak. I have sent bereavement cards, done literature searches for drug information questions, and trained my patients on their blood glucose monitors. I have done all of these things and more because I truly love being a pharmacist.

However, one family has touched me more than all others. This family has endured great pain, yet exudes great strength and love. These parents had three children, the oldest child a son, with two younger daughters, both stricken with cystic fibrosis. Because they were loyal patrons to our pharmacy, our team made sure we were always able to fulfill the medication-related needs of their girls, from their many, many bottles of pancrelipase enzymes to their tobramycin inhalation solution and all the questions in between. Over the years, I grew to admire this strong family for its unrelenting fight to keep the two daughters as healthy as possible. These parents were in our store most days of the week. We met with them early in the morning, late at night, and on weekends. As time went by, the health of their daughters seemed to wax and wane. For the most part, they were healthy; however, periodically, they would develop lung infections that would require extended hospital admissions until they were strong enough to go home. Last summer, their older daughter's health sharply declined. She spent the better part of 3 months in the hospital, climbing the donor list to receive new lungs. I vividly remember researching drug protocols, clinical trials, and natural products, all in an effort to offer her parents a glimmer of hope for some helpful therapeutic option.

I rarely saw the mother during this time when her older daughter was on the wait list. She spent day and night at the hospital. She recalled often forgetting what day it was or the last time she had been home. One night, exhausted and discouraged, she came in to pick up some medication for her younger daughter. I could see she had been crying, her face deep with worry and her skin sallow from the prolonged lack of sunlight. As I finished preparing her prescriptions, I longed for the words to say just the right thing to take some of her worry away. Not only as a pharmacist, but also as a mother of two, I empathized with her feelings of worry and fear. Yet, instead of my offering the first words, she asked how my family was doing. Knowing my older son was entering kindergarten, she questioned me about my concerns for his big step into elementary school. She listened intently and provided me with a source of comfort, an empathetic ear. That night, I realized empathy is not one-sided. As much as I have tried to give to this family through the years, they give back to others in equal measure. They taught me that it is possible to be brave and strong when faced with dire health consequences.

Shortly after this encounter, somewhat unexpectedly, their younger daughter could no longer continue her fight, and passed away. I attended the wake of their young daughter who lost her courageous battle. Hundreds of friends and family lined up to pay their respects long before the service even began. When we entered the funeral home, we were asked to use hand sanitizer and/or surgical masks as her older sister had just received a double lung transplant. The parents stood mightily honoring their daughter who had passed, sympathetically consoling her young friends. Their hearts and minds were filled with fear and worry for their older daughter and her "second chance" at a normal life.

As a community practice faculty member, it is my responsibility to prepare my students to be exemplary community pharmacists. It is not enough for them just to know the facts about medication; they must also consider the humanistic aspect of patient care. Community pharmacists are a presence. They are a reliable and trusted resource for all patients. They provide information on prescription and nonprescription medication, administer immunizations, dispense live-saving and life-altering medication, and provide all of these things with a kind demeanor and a warm smile. Dispensing the right drug, in the right strength, with the right directions to the right patient can be taught. Empathy is a gift. I received this invaluable gift, and I strive to pass it on to my students, our future pharmacists.

A Student's Courage

Lisa Powell, Pharm.D.
Clinician

M any times in the practice, we unintentionally forget about our students and the things that are going on in their personal lives. We are so busy entering orders, checking medications, seeing patients, and counting narcotics that we find it hard to slow down and listen to what our students are saying to us. My friend Brian taught me that it is not only about caring for our patients, but also caring for our students. Here is our story.

I first heard about Brian from one of my colleagues late on a Friday afternoon in April. This preceptor sought my help with a pharmacy student in drug information because I had been a preceptor for students on these rotations in the past. Of course, I was more than willing to help. Then I learned a little about Brian's struggle.

Brian completed his undergraduate degree at the University of North Carolina at Chapel Hill. In March 2009, during his third year at Campbell University School of Pharmacy, he was diagnosed with acute myeloid leukemia. He was sitting in class, where they were going over leukemia. They were going over the symptoms, and Brian was thinking some of the things were happening to him. He had undergone chemotherapy, was in remission, and was completing his pharmacy rotations at Duke University Hospital in Durham, North Carolina, 50 miles from his home. Brian had fallen a little behind in his pharmacy studies. He was teleconferenced into his rotations from his hospital bed, and he had been preparing presentations and studying while undergoing chemotherapy for periods of up to 3 months in the hospital. "Basically, I acted like it was a normal day," said Brian from his hospital bed at Duke University Hospital, where he was on his third round of chemotherapy. "I'd have my chemo going or whatever. I'd set up my desk here. I would talk to my classmates and to Dr. G. And I'd just pound away at my schoolwork. That's just me." He never thought about taking a break from school. "That's the easy way out, to put it plain. I wasn't brought up to do that," he said. "This is a long-term goal I had, and I wasn't going to let sickness or something like that stand in the way of me and my goal.... So I just decided that I was going to keep on going forward." To help him complete his degree, I was to help precept him for his last rotation in May 2010, the month when his other classmates graduated.

I met Brian that following Monday in May 2010, and we instantly bonded. We had gone to the same undergraduate school, and we had a lot in common. We talked about the Carolina Tar Heels, our families, and our church families. Of course, I now see that Brian just had that effect on people. Everyone who met him instantly liked him. His smile was contagious and could be seen in his eyes. Everyone who talked with him walked away feeling better than before because of his infectious positive personality. All the mothers who worked in the pharmacy said that Brian was the type of guy that you would want your daughter to marry. He worked tirelessly for our department, answering questions, completing projects, and writing a newsletter article. He worked so hard, until one day, I told him that he looked very tired. He then told me, "My hemoglobin was only 7 yesterday at my doctor's appointment." I asked him why he came into work that day, and he stated, "I needed to get this done." He failed to report to his rotation assignment only 1 day. "I want to be there, Lisa, but I am in too much pain today" was the e-mail I received from him the next day. He had undergone a bone marrow biopsy the previous day. He was so determined to finish school that he had let only a few people know he was ill.

As we got to know each other, he shared more of his story with me. He was waiting for a match to be found for a bone marrow transplant with the Be the Match Organization. His two sisters had already been tested and were not matches for him. His mother had passed away, and he was estranged from his father. His only hope was to find a match with the Be the Match Organization, and he stated, "It would be difficult because there aren't a lot of black people, African Americans in the registry." As I listened to his story, I instantly realized that someone needed to conduct a bone marrow drive in his honor. It was the first time I realized he felt powerless by not doing anything to find a cure for himself and for others. Part of moving forward for Brian meant getting the word out to minorities about the bone marrow registry. He talked about helping others and educating others about joining the registry; holding a drive would give him the opportunity to live that dream. He was more than willing to share his story and help make it a reality in any way possible. The bone marrow drive in honor of Brian was to be held in June.

The month of May progressed. He continued to be upbeat and positive around everyone while I worked to prepare the logistics for our drive. However, I realized that as I stopped to talk with Brian, he was discouraged and afraid of what lay ahead. He was coming into the pharmacy one day with a smile on his face. I asked him how he was. He paused, took a deep breath, and said, "I am doing okay, Lisa." I could tell he wanted to say more, but he did not want anyone feeling sorry for him. That day was the last time I saw Brian face to face. His leukemia had returned, and he had to go back into the hospital at the end of May.

I kept in touch with Brian while he was in the hospital. We had a bone marrow drive to do in June, and I needed his help to recruit donors. And from his hospital room, helping me recruit is what he did. The local television station came in and did an interview with Brian. "Here I am back in the hospital for another month," joked Brian during his interview. "I would have never guessed at 30 years old I'd come down with leukemia." He interviewed with a local newspaper and participated in a radio talk show at a local university, encouraging folks to come out and get their cheeks swabbed to be included on the registry. Brian was in the medical profession, and I believe he knew that his time was running out. But he kept on working because he knew that it might benefit someone else in the future. "It does no good to sit in here, sad and depressed," said Brian during his interview. He knew that it wasn't just about him, but about his neighbor down the hall who also needed a donor. "Of course, I want a match out of this. Who would be crazy enough to think I wouldn't? But at the same time, I want the next person in the room beside me to get a match as well. I want this for everyone."

The day of our drive, he gave another interview, encouraging folks to come, and come they did. Most of our pharmacy department, now knowing that Brian needed our help, came out to get swabbed or to help run the drive. People who had seen him on television were inspired to come get swabbed as well. I met one man who had heard Brian's story that morning on television and drove 35 miles to be added to the registry. A breast cancer survivor who was touched by Brian's story drove to downtown Greensboro to be tested. She began sobbing when she discovered that, because of her battle with cancer, she could not be added to the registry. She wanted so desperately to help Brian. His story touched a lot of people that day. In total, 100 people were added to the registry.

Despite his tireless work, Brian never found his match and died in September 2010, just 1 month after graduating from pharmacy school.

Now I continue with what we started and have become a volunteer ambassador with the Be the Match Organization. I have told Brian's story at churches and other organizations. His story has influenced at least another 1,500 people to join the registry. Still, I thought we would win in finding him a match, and I miss Brian. We e-mailed each other daily, until he was too sick to do so. When we deal with other medical professionals, it is easy to forget that we are caring for someone's son, mother, or daughter. From Brian, I have learned to slow down and listen, not only to my patients but also to my coworkers.

Will You Be Our Valentine?

Kyle Burghardt, Pharm.D.
Student

A woman in her late 70s was in the hospital for worsening dementia characterized by recent striking out and yelling at her daughter at home. She also had a diagnosis of schizophrenia for more than 30 years. During the first week of her hospital stay, she became known around the unit for making statements such as "Why would I have to take blood pressure medication anymore? I'm cured, my heart is fine!" and "My doctor told me I had diabetes 20 years ago, but she hasn't seen me since then, so how would you or her know if I still have diabetes...I DON'T need to take that diabetes medication, and I'm NOT going to! When I get out of here, I'll be by myself, and I won't take my medication anyways!" She had even thrown her cup of pills on the floor one day out of defiance.

She had been in the hospital for more than 3 weeks and had improved tremendously since that first week. The team had been able to convince her to start taking her blood pressure and diabetes medications voluntarily, and her mental status was also significantly improved. She was generally agreeable during interviews except when discussing her discharge plan. Her daughter would no longer be able to take care of her due to a lack of time and money. We discussed many options with her including assisted living and nursing homes, but she was adamant that she wanted, and was able, to live alone. At the end of each interview, she would become very agitated and annoyed by the lack of progress in her discharge plan and would angrily state, "I've agreed to take my medications, so why won't you just let me live in an apartment by myself? I can take care of myself. I'm trapped in this place." The entire team felt her disgust with the situation but also believed that she no longer had the capacity to live on her own. It seemed as though this patient's progress had hit a wall.

It was Valentine's Day, and the team was interviewing her again. Once more, the interview became strained, and tensions rose as the subject of discharge was addressed. She became so disgusted at one point that she turned in her bed with her arms crossed and refused to face the team. She said, "If you all aren't going to listen to me, why should I even bother talking anyways. It is the same thing EVERY day."

Just as the team was about to end the interview, a social worker asked, "Do you have a valentine for today?"

"No, of course not, and I probably won't since I'm stuck here in this stupid place," she replied with a laugh.

"Well, you never know. There is still plenty of day left," answered the social worker with as much positive energy as she could manage.

Later in the day, as I was working up newly admitted patients and answering drug information questions, I thought perhaps there was a chance for a connection with this unhappy patient that the team was missing. I went to the gift shop to purchase a small Valentine's Day card to give to our patient from the entire team. The card was plain and simple. It had a picture of a cartoon cupid on the front taking aim with his arrow, and on the inside, it read, "Will YOU be my valentine?" When the patient was outside her room participating in a group therapy class where the patients on the unit get together to make their own crafts, I went into her room and placed the card on her pillow. I did not hear anything about it for the rest of the day.

The next morning, during team discussion, we arrived to our most disgruntled patient, and the nurse stated that she was beaming about the valentine.

"This morning, she has been making positive statements about working with the team to get her into a suitable living situation. She even said she would be willing to live in an assisted living facility!" The social worker also said with a surprised look that "Our patient wanted me to thank the team for all of the effort they had given her in the last month."

These positive statements were also present during her interview. When we approached the issue of discharge, our now-pleasant patient was much more open about alternative living situations and did not become agitated or annoyed during the discussion. This was a huge and frankly amazing change from previous interviews!

A few weeks later, the plethora of issues regarding her discharge plan was finally worked out, and she was discharged to an assisted living facility. During the last few weeks, though, she was much more pleasant to the staff, which made life easier for everyone on the unit. In the end, it may seem obvious that this simple act of empathy and altruism was not the main reason for her improvement in health, but it probably played a part. It is hard to say what will happen if you take a few seconds and make a small gesture to a patient. It may not affect your patient's disposition at all, or perhaps it might go a long way to improve the quality of care we are giving to patients and develop a therapeutic alliance. These small gestures are so easy to give that, in some cases, it is worth putting in the extra effort because it may help reach that positive outcome we strive to achieve as health care professionals.

What Drug Is This?

Bonnie A. Labdi, Pharm.D., R.Ph.
Pharmacy Manager

R arely do we come across a patient actually taking a monoamine oxidase inhibitor (MAOI). We learn about all the drug interactions and adverse effects associated with the use of this class of drugs throughout our pharmacy school career. Then, for the majority of us, all of this knowledge is neatly tucked away in our "must-know but will probably never come across" database. I, for one, believe that knowledge never used or reviewed can become buried among all the everyday facts we need to perform well in our professional as well as personal lives. For this reason, I thought a review of an actual situation that occurred with one of my patients would serve as a refresher for those of us who have never had to manage a patient receiving MAOI therapy.

The patient, SW, was a 58-year-old woman whose primary diagnosis was follicular lymphoma, which was in remission. She was admitted on a Friday afternoon through the emergency room to our hospital with a symptomatic urinary tract infection, abdominal pain, and failure to thrive. Her medical history was remarkable for Parkinson disease, hypercholesterolemia, GERD, and follicular lymphoma. She was on a handful of medications for the above-mentioned health problems. Specifically, three of her medications (all for her diagnosis of Parkinson disease) were entacapone, carbidopa-levodopa, and selegiline. Our inpatient pharmacy did not carry selegiline (we rarely had patients taking this or any other MAOI), so the patient's family member was asked to bring in the patient's home supply of it. As (I suspect) is true with many order entry systems, a patient's home medications at our hospital were manually entered in the pharmacy computer as "patient's own med," and because of this, they were quite often not included in the screening for interactions or warnings.

SW's selegiline as well as all of her other medications were continued. She was started on ceftriaxone for her UTI and given intravenous fluids. Over the weekend, the inpatient attending-physician noted that the patient continuously demonstrated a flat affect, which could explain why she was not eating or drinking as she should have. In addition, the family member told the physician that the patient had a remote diagnosis of depression. For this reason, an inpatient psychiatry consult was ordered. The psychiatric service, consisting of a resident and the attending-physician, came on Saturday afternoon and reviewed the patient's history. They discussed (presumably) the patient's condition and her various comorbidities and decided initially to try nonpharmacologic options. On Sunday (according to the written progress note), the resident came by and evaluated the patient. A decision was made to initiate an antidepressant (specifically escitalopram), of which SW received her first dose that day at approximately 2230 hours.

When I came in to round on my patients Monday morning, I noticed that the on-call fellow had been contacted overnight regarding SW's blood pressure, which had peaked at 220/100 around 0130 on Monday. She had received three doses of IV hydralazine by the time I came at around 0700. I quickly reviewed SW's chart and her medical history. Initially, I thought that perhaps she was taking blood pressure medications at home and that the ER physician had left them off her admission orders. However, I discovered that SW had never suffered from hypertension; her blood pressure readings throughout her admission had been in the low 110s over 60s. Then, when I went through all the medications she was currently receiving, I noticed that she had received a dose of escitalopram the night before. I looked at her other medications and saw that she came in on selegiline and entacapone. I wrote an order to discontinue the escitalopram and decrease the IV fluids. I placed a note on the front of the chart saying that any changes in SW's medications would have to be approved by the clinical pharmacy specialist on the primary team (me). Over the next several hours, her blood pressure returned to normal without the need for additional hydralazine.

After much research and a few phone calls, I learned that SW had been on selegiline and entacapone for about 10 years. Both were initiated by her outside neurologist, with whom she had regular follow-up visits to assess her response to treatment as well as to monitor her vital signs. I talked to the psychiatric resident who had started the escitalopram and asked her if she knew what other medications SW was taking. She produced a list of the medications from her progress note. When I asked her if she knew what class of drugs selegiline belonged to, she stated it was an anti-Parkinson drug. When I told her that it was actually an MAOI, she was surprised (mind you, this was a psychiatry resident). Apparently, when the resident discussed SW's case with the attending-physician, she failed to mention that SW was on selegiline, instead stating that SW was taking drugs for her Parkinson disease.

I then talked to the pharmacist who entered the order and asked her if she recognized that selegiline was an MAOI. She admitted that she had forgotten what class of drug it was. When I asked the inpatient pharmacy supervisor why the interaction had not been caught by the pharmacist, she stated that because the selegiline had been entered as the "patient's own med," it had not gone through the interaction screening that normally occurs during order entry. I was alarmed that at least two physicians and a pharmacist, not to mention nursing staff, had missed this interaction (although if a pharmacist doesn't recognize an MAOI, I would not expect that a nurse would either). The on-call fellow also had missed the interaction. He had initiated hydralazine "as needed" for what would clearly be classified as a hypertensive crisis without attempting to figure out the underlying cause.

I am pleased to say that because of this particular incident, the institution where I worked at the time added all the available MAOIs on the market to its pharmacy database. Even though seldom-used drugs like selegiline would not be available in the pharmacy to dispense, the pharmacist would no longer bypass the interaction and warning screening tool to manually enter the "patient's own med." The pharmacist would now choose the actual drug and enter the "patient's own med" in the comments section, and all drugs would be screened appropriately.

As you can see, many opportunities for review and subsequent intervention were missed. That the pharmacist did not remember what class of drugs selegiline belongs to did not really surprise me, but that the pharmacist did not feel the need to look it up did. This incident confirmed for me the old adage that we are never too experienced to learn. Having worked as a clinical pharmacy specialist for almost 10 years, I thought that I had seen it all in terms of inpatient drug therapy. Now that I am a clinical manager, I spend a great deal of time investigating medication errors that have occurred at my institution. I see firsthand the consequences of incorrect assumptions and the resulting misinformed decisions made by pharmacists, nurses, and other health care providers. Because so much emphasis is now placed on getting the medications to the patient in the leanest, most efficient way possible, we have somehow lost a portion of the critical thinking and natural curiosity we once had. We no longer listen to that "inner voice" trying to tell us that we should look up something to double-check ourselves. How long does it really take to verify a dose or to find out some of the less common uses for a particular drug?

I remember that, as a resident, I would look up everything before either writing or processing an order. Obviously, pharmacists cannot look up everything for their entire career. With repetition and experience, however, we also find that we no longer have to lean on the drug information resources as much. Is this always a good thing? At what point do we ask ourselves if being 99 percent sure of something is good enough? Only with our experience and personal knowledge base can we answer questions like these. I have only recently discovered that with experience and time, one of the most important things we need to learn as individuals is what our limitations are. As health care providers, we must also learn how to balance time and safety—getting the task done in an acceptable amount of time, but getting it done right. Moreover, with patients, we have only one chance to get it right, and if this means looking up an unfamiliar drug or taking a little extra time to question an order, I certainly do not think that the patient or his or her caretakers will mind.

In loving memory of Fern A.
Your smile could outshine the brightest star.

Learning Life's Lessons from Unexpected Places

Candis M. Morello, Pharm.D., CDE
Clinical Pharmacy Specialist

Over the years of working as an ambulatory care pharmacist providing MTM Services in outpatient clinics, I have learned more from my patients than I could ever expect to teach them. One example is my time spent in a pharmacist-managed anticoagulation clinic, where I performed point-of-care INR assessments and anticoagulation management. Because most patients had to be monitored every 4–6 weeks for life, I naturally became very familiar with my patients and their families. Learning about my patients' lives was one of my favorite parts of being a pharmacist in this unique setting.

When I first met Sherry, she was in her early 30s, and her daughter, Matilda, was about 9 months old. For such a young woman, Sherry had several serious medical problems, which resulted in frequent hospitalizations and visits to our clinic. As she battled her health issues through the years, she was placed on medications that resulted in significant weight gain and more visits to our clinic because those same drugs interacted with her anticoagulation regimen. She never complained, though—even when she had to be followed weekly. She would just laugh and say, "See ya next week for our date!" Even though her medical situation was complex and her husband traveled 6–9 months of each year, Sherry maintained a positive attitude and focused her energy on being a good mommy and role model for her daughter. While waiting for our appointment, she read books to Matilda and always had a new song or pat-a-cake game to make her daughter laugh. At less than 1 year old, Matilda couldn't walk or talk, yet I noticed how her large, intelligent, brown eyes seemed to take everything in, and I loved the way her sweet smile lit up the whole room. She was clearly a happy baby.

Although Matilda was pensive during the first few visits because I had taken blood from her mommy's finger, she began to warm up to the idea of coming to the clinic. She always had the biggest smile for me when I called them into my exam room, and after a while, she'd say, "Me! Me! Me!," and let me place a Band-Aid on her fake "boo-boo." When Matilda began to say a few words, both Sherry and Matilda surprised me one day when I walked into the clinic and Matilda broke out into a huge grin and exclaimed very proudly, "Hi, Dr. Candis!" With so few words comprising her vocabulary, I couldn't believe she had learned my name—a very precious moment for me.

During our visits, Sherry and I discussed many aspects of her medical condition. As part of our clinic's educational program, I talked with Sherry about the importance of her wearing a medic alert bracelet and teaching Matilda how to dial 911 in case of an emergency. Little did we know that this advice would be put to the test not just once, but twice. At age 2, Matilda made her first emergency call, which saved her mommy's life. Unfortunately, the second time, Sherry was simply too ill for the doctors to help her. Now, Sherry is with the angels above, helping God guide little Matilda's life. Sometimes, Matilda and her dad visit the clinic just to say hello, and Matilda's sunny smile still has that special way of lighting up the entire office.

To this day, I will never forget the way my heart was touched with life's lessons of courage and determination, as shown by Sherry, as well as the unconditional love she displayed for her little girl. Sherry was such a young woman to experience complicated medical problems, but with her positive attitude, she focused on making a loving and happy life for her daughter. In addition, Matilda's brave actions taught me never to underestimate the intelligence of a small child, a lesson I was grateful to have learned when I had my own children. Despite the trauma she has experienced in her short life, Matilda continues to have a sunny attitude, and her big brown eyes are filled with love and wisdom beyond her years. Here I was the one who was supposed to be doing the educating, but in reality, the lessons I learned from Sherry and Matilda will always be sources of inspiration for me.

The Final Sunset

Anna Miszczanczuk Portokalis, Pharm.D.
Student

I now begin the journey that will lead me into the sunset of my life.[1]

These words are part of a final letter addressed to the American people on November 5, 1994. Our 40th president, Ronald Reagan, released a statement revealing the diagnosis of his Alzheimer disease. His diagnosis was not unique; countless numbers had been affected by it long before, and many more have been since that day. What was unique is that the whole world knew. We were all given a chance to reflect, to ponder, to grieve. But what did it mean to grieve?

The expression of grief is highly individual, expressed by many people in many ways. Is it possible that there really are five stages, or perhaps only five stages, of grief: denial, anger, bargaining, depression, and acceptance?[2] Who experiences these stages, and how long do we linger in them?

The stages are not always unique to those who have lost through death or only to those who love the one lost. To some degree, compassionate pharmacists will experience at least one of them with several patients, whether consciously aware of it or not. Some will never visit more than one stage or spend more than 20 seconds in any particular stage; others may experience all five of them in one patient encounter or in several years of caring for the same patient. In doing so, these pharmacists will demonstrate understanding, tolerance, and empathy for their patients throughout the course of illness.[3] Others will visit the stages vicariously, offering emotional support to family members and friends of their patients.

Whatever the situation may be, compassionate pharmacists possess an empathetic soul that longs to grieve with those under their care. Denial, anger, bargaining, depression, and acceptance are no strangers to the doorway of a pharmacist's heart and mind. Whenever we, together with our patients, face the uncertainty of a diagnosis, stages of disease progression, caregiver burdens, or dying and death, we uphold the Oath of a Pharmacist.[4] Most notably, we consider the welfare of humanity and relief of suffering our primary concern, often achieved by sharing the burden of grief.

I was reminded of this fact in one of my first patient encounters. I was completing my third year of pharmacy school in an outpatient clinic, where I shadowed both pharmacists and doctors. Part of the experience required me to sit in on visits of patients, as the doctor examined them.

"Doctor," said the salt and pepper–haired lady after shuffling into the small office with her white-haired husband. She sat down in the chair next to the doctor's, and her husband seated himself on the examination table with a sigh. She continued, "He seems to be forgetting things lately."

"What kinds of things?" the doctor asked.

"Well, you know..." she continued. "Things like faces. He doesn't recognize the faces of people we knew 30 or 40 years ago. We ran into some old neighbors, and he didn't recognize them."

"Well, faces change a lot in 30 years. I probably wouldn't recognize them either," the doctor said chuckling. "What other things is he forgetting?"

"Well," she said, pausing to think, "He took a wrong turn the other day coming home from our daughter's house and started heading for the house we lived in 10 years ago."

"How often does this happen?" asked the doctor.

"Only the one time," replied the wife.

"Oh, leave me alone on that one," interrupted the husband. "She won't let me forget it, so believe me that it was only the one time."

"I see," said the doctor with a smile. Turning to the husband, he asked a series of three rapid-fire questions:

"What year is it?"

"2010" was the reply.

"What did you have for breakfast?"

"Oatmeal."

"Who is the president?"

"Michelle Obama." Then he let out with a small, sheepish chuckle, "I mean Mister Obama."

"That's not funny," chided the wife.

Turning to the doctor, she wiped some tears. "This is really hard for me because he really is forgetting a lot of things...like where he puts things. I can never find things after he uses them because they're always in the wrong place when he's done."

"OK," said the doctor. "Let's order some tests...we'll start with vitamin and electrolyte levels..." He went on describe what he would like to see evaluated in the elderly man seated on the examination table.

"Oh, thank you!" exclaimed the wife.

Not soon after, the doctor finished the physical examination, and the elderly couple was off to the pharmacy outpatient waiting area. The doctor turned to me and looked straight into my eyes.

"You know, sometimes it's the one complaining that the spouse is forgetful who is really the one becoming forgetful."

I struggled to wrap my mind around what he had just said. Could it really be that she, rather than he, needed the follow-up tests?

Of all the patient encounters I have experienced in my clinical practice development, this one stands out in my mind as having the greatest impact. As I was observing the initial conversations and interactions in the room during that visit, I felt sad for the elderly man. This couldn't be happening to him. He appeared to be physically fit, despite his age. He was well dressed, and his hair was still thick, wavy, and well groomed. He even flashed what I imagined to be a devilish smile that would have melted all the girls' hearts in his younger years. In fact, he still had the twinkle in his eye to match. Obviously, his wife must have been mistaken and was just being overly cautious. Denial had taken over my mind.

Those thoughts quickly changed gears. What was life going to be like for him if he had dementia? Alzheimer disease? Would he know what was happening? Could he tell if it was progressing? How long would it be before he forgot everyone around him? How long would he live? These thoughts quickly filled my mind as the doctor ran through the list of lab tests he was ordering. They were the questions of a pharmacy student experiencing the stage of depression. Although short-lived and only superficial, sadness and numbness were in my heart.

"At least he has a loving wife who will look after him," I thought just as soon as I processed the feelings of depression. In my mind, I was bargaining with the disease that was surely besetting his brain and sense of self. Surely no disease could stand up to the strength this woman displayed. It would just have to give up and go elsewhere. It was as though her presence, her love, and her care could stop the progression of the disease and even give back what it might have already erased.

But then I mulled that last thought: "what it might have already erased." What a horrible disease; what a horrible life—no, death—sentence. I had already chosen Alzheimer disease as the diagnosis and claimed it as my emotional punching bag. I was angry at it and at how it provides no warning when it hits; how it will not allow us to definitively diagnose it; how it prevents us from knowing how to avoid it; how it evades being cured; how it can erase a beautiful mind to the point where one cannot recognize one's own reflection in a mirror. It ravages the mind, soul, and body, removing the person and leaving only a shell. Why was it so cruel?

Almost immediately, as I processed my thoughts of anger, I felt sad again, only now for his wife. She was clearly headed down a difficult road, having to care for her husband. He would no longer be her equal partner, her protector, her provider. She would resume the role of nurturer—a role she had played decades ago when her children were young—only now, it would be for her husband. It looked as though she already took on the role with the love and care she displayed at the visit moments earlier. He would have someone to look after him, and it seemed to be the best anyone could ask for. It would work out in the end, somehow, and doctors, nurses, social workers, and pharmacists would all be there to give their support. I had come to accept that the outcome would be all right.

Although not aware of it at the time, in one brief 20-minute visit, I had experienced, in some capacity, the stages of grief in the context of an Alzheimer diagnosis and its progression leading to death. I was able to understand the breadth, if not the depth, of loss and grief. To say I now understood grief because of this encounter would be an injustice to those who have loved, lost, and grieved. My experience may be comparable to a reflection in a mirror—a representation, but not the real thing. However, the emotions were still real, and I felt as though I had lost something—or someone.

Without minimizing my feelings, emotions, and thoughts regarding what had happened with the man during this visit, I found that it was the comment the doctor had made to me after the couple left that had me feeling even more sadness for the wife than I had for the husband. What if he was right? What if she is the one with early stages of dementia? Is she on that downward spiral of Alzheimer disease? How sad to go through your days forgetting things, blaming others for your mistakes, being driven mad by what you perceive to be others' misperceptions. How sad to have an illness and not even recognize it. Does she have a nurturer in her life to care for her?

I hope that the doctor is wrong on this one, and that neither husband nor wife is in the early stages of dementia and Alzheimer disease. Perhaps all of their worries can be attributed to that good old scapegoat, "the senior moment," and neither one is experiencing the final sunset.

It is moments like these that remind pharmacists to consider the welfare of humanity and relief of suffering our primary concern.[4] As we work alongside a team of medical professionals to provide the best medical care possible, we must also provide the most nurturing and compassionate care possible. We must demonstrate understanding, tolerance, and empathy as we seek to provide care and healing physically, mentally, and emotionally.[3] Compassionate pharmacists seek answers to the questions that are so often asked when a disease is diagnosed and imposed on a person as a life—and death—sentence. "What will life be like for…?" "How long will it be before…?" "Who will care for…?" We will cycle through uncertainties, diagnoses, disease progression, caregiver burdens, losses, and grief with our patients and their families. As pharmacists, we will also face denial, anger, bargaining, depression, and finally acceptance as our patients and their loved ones confront illness and death. It is acceptance of the diagnosis that allows us each to act, do our jobs well, and help create the most beautiful sunset possible.

1. PBS/WGBH Educational Foundation: American Experience [homepage on the Internet]. Available at www.pbs.org/wgbh/americanexperience/features/primary-resources/reagan-alzheimers/. Accessed April 30, 2011.
2. Grief.com [homepage on the Internet]. Kübler-Ross E, Kessler D. The Five Stages of Grief. Available at grief.com/the-five-stages-of-grief/. Accessed April 30, 2011.
3. Wagner J, Goldstein E. Pharmacist's role in loss and grief. Am J Hosp Pharm 1977;34:490–2.
4. Oath of a Pharmacist. American Association of Colleges of Pharmacy. Adopted 2007. Available at www.aacp.org/resources/academicpolicies/studentaffairspolicies/documents/oathofapharmacist2008-09.pdf. Accessed April 30, 2011.

At the Counter, Bedside, and Beyond

Care in a Variety of Settings

*If you find it in your heart to care for
somebody else, you will have succeeded.*

Maya Angelou

*The miracle is not that we do this work,
but that we are happy to do it.*

Mother Teresa

Life-Changing Days in the Trauma ICU

Jennifer M. Belavic, Pharm.D., FASCP
Clinician, Trauma ICU

An 80-year-old man was transferred from an outside hospital as a level 2 trauma patient after slipping and falling on ice in late December 2009. He complained of some facial pain and neck pain. His GCS was 15 upon admission. He was diagnosed with a type II odontoid fracture, multiple left facial fractures, and left periorbital ecchymosis. He was placed in a C-collar, and consults were made to the spine, facial trauma, and ophthalmology services. He was then transferred to the neurological step-down unit to monitor his airway and neurologic status.

In the early morning hours of his fourth hospital day, he was transferred to the trauma ICU due to respiratory distress and was then intubated and sedated. This is when I first saw his name on my census, and I realized that I had known this man my whole life.

He was then extubated, but that failed because he was unable to manage his secretions and clear his airways. He was reintubated. At this point, the plan of care was determined to go in one of two directions. The first plan was conservative management for 7 days with antibiotics, pulmonary toileting, nutrition, and extubation. If his extubation failed, he would then be reintubated and scheduled for a tracheostomy and percutaneous feeding tube placement, with the eventual goal of being transferred to a long-term acute care facility, followed by a skilled nursing facility. The second direction of care included conservative treatment for 7 days and plans for extubation as well. But, if his extubation failed this time, he would not be reintubated, and he would receive comfort measures only. These plans were discussed with the family.

And finally, on day 7, the day after Christmas, a conversation was held with the family to make the decision to provide the patient with comfort measures only. This decision was based on the fact that he would need a tracheostomy and a PEG tube placed, with eventual transfer to a nursing home, and the need for long-term healing from his C2 fracture. According to his wife and son, these measures were not what he would have wanted, and they did not want to see him suffer. Later that evening, the patient died.

Working in the trauma ICU, I see this situation occur over and over again. I have witnessed the hard decisions and suffering that families go through to make the decision of making their loved ones comfortable and watching them pass away. I am part of that multidisciplinary team that provides end-of-life care. Some patients who go through this affect me more than others. But this patient was different. This is one of the many patients that I will remember for the rest of my life. This was a man I had known personally my whole life. He watched me grow up. I went to school with his son. Both of our families belong to the same church. I know this family very well. Walking into the unit in the morning, preparing for rounds, and getting to know my patients are normal for me. But, for anyone, when you see a name you know, you see the family in the patient's room, a family you have known your whole life, and it shakes you to your core.

Every day, I make decisions as a pharmacist for the best care of many patients. And being part of the team that makes decisions about someone I know makes my job a little harder. I know that being the friendly face that the family knows makes a big difference, even if I am "just" the pharmacist on the team. Doctor after doctor, white coat after white coat, nurse after nurse: they move in and out of that room. Each provides information, answers questions, and offers suggestions to the plan of care, which all can be confusing and overwhelming for a patient's family. But the moment a familiar face appears in the room, the white coat disappears, the confusion decreases, and the caring that has been there the whole time is more pronounced.

I show empathy every day. Working in the trauma ICU opens my eyes to the importance of life. Not all of the patients who come through the front door are people who were sick originally. They were living their life one day, and the next, they were experiencing a life-changing accident or trauma. Granted, there are some people I can look at, hear their story and mechanism of injury, and can't help but think: "What were they thinking?" and "Why did they do something so stupid like that?" But then there are the majority of the patients that I can feel extreme empathy for, and I do everything in my power to fix them, tune them up, and make them better. There are joyous days in the trauma ICU when the patient gets well enough to transfer to the general medicine floors, or even go off to rehab. But there are also days that upset you, depress you, make you question if life is fair.

There will be that day in your career when you take care of someone that you know. And no matter what the outcome is, you will be affected. As for me, I knew the moment I saw his name in my census that my life would be changed forever. And I know that, from that moment on, my ability to practice pharmacy changed for the better.

Care and Empathy

Brenda T. Smith, R.Ph., PIC, M.S.
Pharmacist

During a regular workweek, the pharmacy always had the pleasure of a visit from a patient, JU, a white man, 50 years old, slightly heavy in build. JU was very friendly to all the staff, easy going, well-educated with a master's degree in engineering, divorced with two children. As one of our patients, JU was a very personable individual and was well-liked by all the pharmacy staff. He was well-informed, interested in learning new information, and inquisitive about new medications. He often would come to the pharmacy to inquire about medications that could be of assistance to him in alleviating his headaches, or that might be causing his hearing loss. He had been on tramadol and alprazolam for several years. We discussed the use of tramadol and the possible correlation of it with his hearing loss. He was then switched to Darvocet-N-100 to alleviate the headaches. We discussed the differences in drugs within the same class for his anxiety disorder. He questioned the differences in changing clonazepam to alprazolam or lorazepam to get the maximum benefit. He never rushed; moreover, he showed a great interest in each of the pharmacy staff, joked with each of us, and kept us abreast of the news. He kept us informed on the local news and the newest developments about the U.S. president. We discussed each of our family situations. JU, who was divorced, had a lot of personal problems with his ex-wife and dealing with her breast cancer, as well as financial difficulties. As the pharmacist on duty, I was able to get to know a great deal about JU. We often discussed his medications and the symptoms he was experiencing with or without his medications. He would read about a specific drug and then would speak with me about the potential of trying it for his headaches or anxiety. He listened intently and talked to his doctor about the new information he had learned from our talks, often trying different medications to alleviate his symptoms. He tried all antidepressants in the SSI class. Once a medication was effective, he remained adherent to his medication therapy.

One Friday evening, March 14, 2008, JU came into the pharmacy and stood over the counter from me very quietly. His face was flushed. I spoke with him and he told me that he had experienced an episode earlier that evening and was unable to speak or hold the phone in his right hand. I immediately asked him to check his blood pressure with our monitor. He remained withdrawn, quiet, and unable to communicate effectively with me. He could not complete an entire sentence, and often he paused without finishing the sentence, trying to find the right expression that he wanted to say. His words were slurred, and his sentences were incomprehensible. He had repeat episodes of dysphagia, unable to get out the words he wanted. This would clear and then occur again. His blood pressure was very high, 150/100 mm Hg. We waited and then remeasured his blood pressure. Again, it read extremely high, and I advised him to go to the emergency department. JU hesitated, gave excuses about going later if he continued to have episodes or felt cloudy headed. I offered to take him, and he refused. Not taking "no" for an answer, and explaining the gravity of the situation, I insisted on calling the rescue squad. At that point, he agreed to go directly to the emergency department, driving himself. I called ahead to the emergency department, explaining the severity of his situation, his appearance, and his actions while at the pharmacy so that they would be waiting for him when he arrived. They did an EKG and an x-ray immediately. His blood pressure was 180/115 mm Hg. JU was admitted for observation. The next morning, JU experienced another episode of confusion, during which he could not speak or communicate with the nurse. A CT scan was performed that showed reduced blood flow to the left side of the brain with no hemorrhage. On Sunday, March 16, 2008, JU lost the ability to speak again, and could not understand what anyone was saying. An MRI was ordered that Monday. It showed a moderate stroke to the left temporal lobe and reduced flow to the left carotid artery. As a result, a bilateral carotid artery study was performed to both sides of his neck. The left side showed 100% blockage with no flow noted in the left internal carotid artery, and the right side was normal, with no significant disease. I was allowed copies of the patient's history and physical examination on admission, CT scan, carotid artery study, and discharge summary by JU.

The pharmacy had not seen or spoken to JU in several months, not since he had been admitted to the hospital. I kept abreast of his situation with his father and of the severity of JU's condition. After months of absence, JU reappeared at the pharmacy with his father. I was so relieved to see that he had survived the traumatic ordeal. He was not as talkative, and often he showed signs of short-term memory loss and communication problems. He still experienced slurred speech. He could not remember the visit to the pharmacy or what had happened to him upon admission. JU could not complete an entire sentence. He was mentally and physically fatigued, and he could not stand for long periods. He had to sit while waiting on his medications. He was not as patient and jovial; he was now quiet and withdrawn. Depression and anxiety continually added to his communication problem. He spoke of his frustration about the inability to say what he was thinking, and it had caused considerable sleep problems. The stroke and hearing loss both compounded his communication and impeded his ability to overcome this adversity. Over time, JU returned regularly to the pharmacy. He seemed accepting of his condition and never dwelled on the negative. JU continued to be a welcome sight at the pharmacy. I recently ran into JU and immediately remembered the traumatic event. I asked him to comment on it. "I am thankful to be alive after my ordeal; I try to be positive and realize that things could have been worse. I feel that I am lucky and that if I never get any better than I am today, that is OK." I am so grateful to know I made a life-saving decision for JU and that he is still with us today.

As a pharmacist, I know that my interactions with JU through listening intently, observing, and reacting to his responses—and not taking "no" for an answer—contributed to a positive outcome. As JU's pharmacist, I cared about him, showed a commitment to his health, and let him know I was always there if he needed me. JU's first response to his initial episode was to come to the pharmacy. It has been 3 years since this event occurred. JU is a viable, likable person. He is accepting of his condition and enjoys life to the fullest. I am a much richer person for knowing JU, and I am grateful he came to me when he needed assistance. He has shown me how important it is to know your patients, interact with them, and look for minute differences in their behavior. JU's outlook gave me renewed hope in my ability to serve the community to improve the health of, and ensure optimal outcomes for, my patients.

Serving Those Who Have Served

Brandon Sucher, Pharm.D., CDE, AE-C
Educator

W hen I hear news of our military serving abroad, I find myself reflecting on my time spent serving the veterans at the West Palm Beach Veterans Affairs Medical Center (WPB VAMC). It was here that I gained a greater appreciation for veterans' service to our country. And it was here that my approach to pharmacy practice changed. Instead of applying evidence-based medicine to achieve therapeutic goals and optimize patient care, my approach shifted to listening to patients and applying what I call *situational patient care*.

Upon arrival to my first pharmacy practice faculty position with Palm Beach Atlantic University (PBA), I was eager to enter a practice site where I could use my literature evaluation skills and apply lessons learned from direct patient care experiences. During my primary care specialty residency, I had numerous opportunities to apply evidence-based medicine to help patients achieve therapeutic goals and optimize patient care for patients with hypertension, dyslipidemia, and diabetes mellitus (DM). Although my residency training did not specifically include patient care responsibilities at a VA, my residency experiences equipped me with the skills to provide patient care services in the primary care pharmacotherapy clinics at the WPB VAMC, which focused on helping patients achieve therapeutic goals for hypertension, dyslipidemia, and DM.

Seven years and more than 5,000 patient visits seemed to go by in the blink of an eye. I quickly learned that optimizing patient care was more about listening to patients and less about medication adjustments. Early in my practice, one of my most challenging patients was referred by a colleague. "Was this some sort of hazing or initiation?" I thought. This patient's type 2 DM had progressed to needing insulin therapy. The patient's refusing to eat more than one meal a day resulted in an insulin regimen of maintenance insulin and once-daily mealtime insulin. Insulin adjustments rarely resulted in any significant improvements in A1C lab results. Forget about the opportunity to review a self-monitoring blood glucose log. His bipolar disorder added complexity because he seemed to care very little about controlling his DM, even though other health care providers continued to progressively amputate his lower limbs.

It took a few years for me to really listen to him and understand his perspective. Over time, he shared details of his combat experiences when his fellow soldiers didn't survive. He felt he should have died with them. When you don't think you should have survived the Vietnam War, preventing complications from uncontrolled DM is a low priority. My approach to patient care changed from a compliance model to an empowerment model. In other words, instead of trying to influence patients to adhere to evidence-based treatment recommendations, my patient education focused on preparing patients to make their own informed decisions about their treatment. Often, I found myself applying a balance of these two approaches as I developed a perception of a patient's education preferences. Ultimately, my appointments with this patient became times of active listening during his manic episodes while trying to make him laugh during his episodes of depression. Our visits often ended with him saying, "Thanks for listening, chaplain."

"Happy Birthday, Captain!" I exclaimed as I called back another one of my patients, one of the most enthusiastic. I always did my best to look for recent birth dates in each patient's profile before seeing them in my office. I began seeing this patient during a time when metformin and second-generation sulfonylureas were first choice on the VA formulary for patients with type 2 DM. Insulin was the next step for most patients, as the use of glitazones was non-formulary. This particular patient was referred for dyslipidemia management because his type 2 DM was well controlled with metformin. Previous health care providers had avoided the use of sulfonylureas in him because he had a documented allergy to sulfa (rash) in his profile. I also noticed he had diarrhea as a documented adverse drug reaction to metformin. Our initial visits focused on reaching his LDL cholesterol goal, which was easily achieved by titrating his statin dose.

As our relationship progressed, he asked me if there was anything else he could use to treat his type 2 DM. He looked unusually depressed that day. I introduced the option of insulin, but he was afraid he would lose his fishing boat captain license if he started insulin. A subsequent visit revealed that he was wearing diapers during his fishing boat tours, and it was embarrassing when he had diarrhea on his tours. At the time, there was enough literature to support a careful trial of a sulfonylurea in patients with allergies to other sulfa drugs. We agreed on the calculated risk of a trial of glipizide instead of metformin. He assured me that he would discontinue glipizide and report to the emergency room if he experienced shortness of breath or a rash. He returned glowing. "I can't wait to show you my blood glucose log!" He had replaced metformin with glipizide, with no adverse effects to the glipizide, and his self-monitoring of blood glucose reflected good glycemic control.

I tried to hide my skepticism because I had already seen too many falsified blood glucose logs from other patients. "These look within range. Let's see how the A1C looks." I was elated to discover his fasting blood glucose and A1C from the lab results reflected good glycemic control. It seemed like a simple intervention at the time, but after that intervention, he raved about me to other patients in the waiting room. "That's him," he would say, pointing at me just before getting up to walk with me from the waiting room to my office. It was somewhat embarrassing. I tried to explain to him that I really shouldn't reschedule him since the VA's policy was to discharge patients from the pharmacotherapy clinics after achieving therapeutic goals. He convinced me to reschedule him for "medication review" appointments every 3–6 months to see how things were going. Most of the visits were focused on listening to his fishing stories, and he invited me to join him when he didn't have tours booked. But these meetings allowed me to update his medications and ask him what questions he had for me. One question about the results of a bone mineral density scan earlier in the year led to catching an overlooked diagnosis of osteoporosis, which his physician promptly treated after a simple communication of the results with him.

Listening to and empathizing with veterans led to the development of trust and lasting relationships that ultimately enhanced patient care. Helping patients understand and navigate through an organized but complicated health care system was an added priority for me. Over time, these relationships progressed to friendships, and I found myself with a mortgage broker and a fishing buddy among my patients. I tried to learn as many of their names as possible so that I could call patients from the waiting room to my office with eye contact and a simple nod of the head or by gently placing my hand on the shoulder of a veteran who had fallen asleep while waiting.

I have a great deal of respect for our veterans, and it was a privilege to serve and advocate for those who have safeguarded our nation both in peace and in war. I enjoyed seeing students develop a passion for caring for veterans, and I'm pleased to see several PBA alumni seek out residencies and pharmacy positions within the VA health care system. I'm also proud to have a brother with more than 20 years of service in the Air Force and proud to have been part of an organization dedicated to serving those whose service to our country has earned the love, respect, and admiration of a grateful nation.

The "Expert" Witness

Richard J. Artymowicz, Pharm.D., FCCP, BCPS
Clinician/Director

I was introduced to the idea of the medical expert witness during my residency. My residency preceptor had earned a reputation among the physicians in the county as an "expert" in drugs (we would call it pharmacotherapy today). On the recommendation of one of the local physicians, a prominent malpractice attorney used my preceptor as an expert witness on a case. The case went well, word of mouth spread, and over the years, my preceptor had built a nice side business. I found all of this pretty alluring as a resident. I already had great respect for the man just from watching him practice his craft at the hospital. I could only imagine him in a courtroom, calmly and confidently explaining the nuances of the pharmacotherapy in the case, and the feeling he must have at the end knowing that he helped vindicate a fellow health care provider wrongly accused or helped a patient heal in another way after being harmed by a careless physician. That was a feeling I knew I wanted to experience.

After residency, my "expert witness" fantasies, with me saving the day with some obscure piece of knowledge (and getting a nice one-liner in on the cross-examining attorney), faded. I was busy building my own practice in another state, and there weren't any malpractice attorneys in town. My first opportunity came 3 years into my career, and quite by chance. A friend of a college roommate of mine was an attorney in yet another state and had mentioned to my friend that he needed an expert for this wrongful death suit he was defending. So I got the call. And then I got two printer paper boxes full of medical records delivered. And then I got scared! So an emergency phone call went out to my mentor from residency, and he calmly explained to me what I had gotten into.

There is no course in pharmacy school about being an expert witness. If there were, I wonder who would teach it. As I learned, physicians often charge upward of $2,000 an hour just for record review.

Today, pharmacists will get $250–$1,000 an hour, depending on their experience. Even though tuition has gone up, I don't see the schools laying out this kind of coin for adjunct faculty. But fortunately, my Sensei was willing to guide his grasshopper through this. And I got lucky the first time. I found something in the medical record that the attorneys hadn't spotted, and even though this had nothing to do with the original question posed, they used it to win their case. That daydream was starting to come true, and I didn't have to go to court or even do a deposition…. "This might be easier than it looks."

Nothing could have been further from the truth. About a year later, the same practice called me about another case. It seemed like a slam dunk on the phone, but this time it was a plaintiff case. The attorney did a great job of practicing his opening statement on me when he pitched the case. It involved the alleged overprescribing of painkillers, and the patient really seemed to have been taken advantage of by the physician. I felt like I knew the kind of physician this person was, because I thought I knew the type from physicians that I had worked with. Careless, apathetic, outdated…the kind of person that deserved to be taught a lesson. I thought I was going to help someone and make a difference by maybe helping to expose the negligence. This was the wrong line of thinking to pursue. Expert witnesses need to focus on a single issue and give their opinions (which should be based on experience and supported by literature and accepted practice) to the attorneys and then let the attorneys use this information to defend their case. Nothing more. I was about to receive a painful lesson on this.

This case wasn't going away with me offering advice on the phone. After I reviewed the records (there were obvious prescribing irregularities) and discussed my opinions with the attorney, a deposition with the defense attorney was set. Emergency phone call No. 2! As my now-friend explained, the first part of the deposition would be a series of questions to establish that you were indeed an expert. I was told to expect questions like "Where did you go to medical school?" and statements like "So you're not a real doctor then." The attorney would want to know how often I worked as an expert witness (do this too frequently and it can become a point of attack for the other attorneys). The second part would actually be questions about the case, and oh, by the way, the attorney will try to manipulate what you say to his favor, so be concise and confident, and for the love of Pete, don't inject any emotion! Because the case was out of state, the attorney I was working for only listened in on the phone; the defense attorney (also out of state) came to my office with a stenographer. So I had no experience doing this, no support person in the room,...and no chance.

Actually, it wasn't as bad as it could have been. I did manage to get my point across and not become too defensive when challenged, but it went down as one of the worst experiences of my life (and remember, I didn't do anything wrong...I was the expert!). At one point, the defense attorney had me so flustered that I blurted out a totally incorrect statement. The second most embarrassing thing about the whole process was reading the transcript and having to see that mistake in print. The MOST embarrassing part was reading transcripts from defense experts pointing it out! The daydream had become a nightmare. But it really didn't end that bad. The case was settled out of court (sparing the client and me court testimony), but I had decided that the expert witness business was not for me.

That was, until my mentor called about 10 years later and explained that one of the firms he worked for really needed a pharmacist and that he wasn't right for it, but he thought that I was. Partly because he asked, and partly because I felt like I needed a chance at redemption, I took the case. This one involved a hospital patient, and we were defending the physician. I felt more confident this time. I was older and more experienced, and although I felt like the physician had acted justly, I stayed morally grounded without any delusions of teaching someone I didn't know a lesson. The deposition had to be done by phone again, but this time, I was prepared. I was confident and concise, and I wasn't fazed in the least when my knowledge, integrity, or status as an expert was challenged. I wanted to do a good job, and I would have been disappointed if the physician I was helping defend was found negligent, but by not getting too emotional, I did a much better job. This time, it was me pointing out errors in the plaintiff's experts' depositions.

Since then, I've gotten two more calls to be an expert. One case was just a "what do you think" call, and the other finally cemented for me what this is all about. After reviewing the records (it was another defense case), I called the attorney and recommended that he try to settle or find another expert because there was no way I could defend what the physician did. He took a third option and called me two more times, asking me to "look at it another way" or, "if I could just say it this way instead, then he'd have something to work with." Hey, he was just doing his job, but any remnants of the original daydream about saving the day, upholding justice, and getting zingers in on unsuspecting attorneys were pretty much gone after that. The expert witness business had been exposed for what it was...a business.

My perspective on being an expert witness is just that, mine. Pharmacists can make great expert witnesses, and believe me, they are needed to help keep the checks and balances of malpractice cases in order. But for those of you considering this kind of work, you will be well served if you do the following: (1) find a true expert to mentor you through the process because there is no substitute for this, (2) don't get emotionally invested in any case, and (3) do it for the right reasons. If your motivation is financial, get on a speaker's bureau. But if you want to help people, have thick-enough skin to endure the depositions, and have a true-enough moral compass to avoid persuasion, you'll find satisfaction...and perhaps that elusive opportunity for the one-liner to the attorney.

Advocating for the Patient with Pain Using Knowledge and Empathy

Karen F. Marlowe, Pharm.D., BCPS, CPE
Clinician

I began my career in pharmacy practice in a pediatric intensive care unit, which included children after open heart surgery. It was my distinct pleasure over 6 years to develop pharmacotherapy services in this unit with the intensivists and surgeons using a collaborative model of care. Our pharmaceutical care model included pharmacokinetic dosing and antibiotic monitoring as well as pain management. In the intensive care environment, adequate pain management was always a significant struggle between the patient's cardiovascular stability, progress with ventilator weaning, and ability to regain mobility. As pharmacists, our assessment of pain and need for treatment can be in contrast to the priorities of the rest of the team. Our unique perspective allows us to see when the pharmacology of individual analgesics or sedatives may be appropriate in an individual patient situation. In other situations, side effects may necessitate using lower doses or adding another agent such as a laxative or antihistamine to allow the use of an analgesic. We have the ability to create a therapy plan that can adapt to the changing condition of the patient, and by putting all of our prior experience into play, we can give our patients the best possible experience. A pharmacist has the opportunity to be an advocate for the patient by managing the patient's pharmacotherapy. If we aren't the leaders in pain management, pain and sedation can get lost in other priorities.

In my first year of practice, we cared for an infant who had deteriorated significantly during her time in the ICU. She had never fully recovered from her surgery for a congenital heart defect. She was only a few months old, and during her stay in the ICU, she experienced many complications. After being in the unit for several weeks, she developed sepsis and was struggling with multiple organ dysfunction. A feature of my practice is a close association with patients and their families during their ICU stay. Parents spend many hours at their child's bedside. As a clinician, I find it difficult to see the child in such a helpless position and to observe the parents' struggle to support their child through this type of illness and the complications it brings. Parents are distraught at their child's appearance, which commonly involves the ventilator, chest tubes, and several intravenous lines and central catheters. Many of these children are quite edematous.

After developing sepsis and organ dysfunction, this particular infant required three vasopressors and developed such severe edema that her extremities were seeping fluid. She had many central lines and chest tubes. Despite the gravity of her situation, she was not given any continuous pain medication. The instability of her blood pressure was provided as the rationale for not using routine opioids. Day after day, I pushed the issue with several attending physicians and her surgeon. Through the week, she continued to become clinically less stable. I voiced with the team during rounds that perhaps unmanaged pain was a reason for her lack of clinical improvement. I believe that speaking for the patient in this setting and promoting the use of analgesia is part of our role within the health care team. It is also a moral imperative. How can we as health care professionals let a human being suffer?

While it is fairly easy to intervene regarding a drug level or microbiologic culture results, intervening on the behalf of patients who cannot speak regarding their pain is like moving a brick wall. Many clinicians still put pain behind other issues on their priority list. In their minds, it is just not as important. We discuss it on rounds, but if you are not sitting with that patient each day or talking with his or her family, it does not make the top of the priority list. Finally, I tried suggesting that her untreated pain could be the source of her instability with another one of the ICU physicians, the attending who was in charge of the unit for the week. To be quite honest, I am not sure he believed there was a connection between her pain and her clinical situation. He did believe, however, that she was so close to death that we should ensure her comfort through continuous opioids, so he ordered a fentanyl drip. I remember delivering it to her bedside and then standing with her nurse as she started the drip—knowing that I had done the right thing for this child. Within hours, her blood pressure stabilized, and by the end of the day, she had been weaned to one vasopressor. Her condition continued to improve, and within 2 weeks, she left the ICU. I remember this patient and her family almost every day.

The experience of caring for this patient and others like her taught me, like no textbook could, that untreated pain has physiologic consequences. Pain can be a symptom, but as clinicians, we must approach it with the mind-set of managing a disease state. By placing it on our priority list, we are able to advocate for the patient. While the clinical decision-making for the symptom of pain is about making short-term choices for one or two doses, a disease-state approach is about pharmacotherapy planning and monitoring. We choose medications and other therapies to try to manage the patient's pain for the long-term outcome. Our goal should not be about the next pain score but about the goals of the patient and the family: what is it that they want from their therapy?

As pharmacists, we must consider all parts of the plan and work with all members of the team—even if we have to educate the team members about pain to bring them on board. Nonpharmacologic interventions are part of the plan. Prevention of side effects is always considered in the pain management plan; also considered are the patient's other conditions, which thereby makes for an individualized plan. Because of this infant's experience, we were incorporated into the multidisciplinary care meetings held to coordinate care for these complex cases. At a smaller level, my recommendation pertaining to analgesics and sedation was much more likely to be accepted. This added responsibility encouraged me to seek formal training in pain management.

I learned so much from caring for this infant. She inspired me to learn more about pain management and individualized approaches to pain and palliative care. I have continued to learn throughout my career, and I now share that knowledge as a Certified Pain Educator. One of the most basic needs of patients, throughout the life spectrum, is to be comfortable. As a health care provider, I continue to struggle to balance this basic desire with the risks associated with all classes of pain medications. I find this requires advocacy, working with patients to titrate medications to their pain, manage their side effects, and educate them and their family regarding their therapies. The hardest teaching point for patients and their families to understand is, "We cannot eliminate your pain, but we can make it tolerable."

I believe this area of therapy will have a huge impact on almost every area of practice during the next decade as the population ages. Many of the prevalent disorders—such as diabetes, coronary heart diseases, and chronic kidney disease—have pain disorders that go along with them—for example, diabetic neuropathy or peripheral vascular disease. In addition, many of our veterans are returning with chronic pain syndromes. The pharmacist should not only be able to provide expertise in this area, but should also serve as an advocate for the patient. All patients in pain deserve to have someone who is knowledgeable about their condition and medication and someone who is in a position to help them understand their disease management. As I learned from the infant in the ICU, pain should be managed with the same respect we give any disease state.

Patient Care: Delivered Aurally

Lindsay Davison, Pharm.D.
Drug Information Specialist

The federal government is not the first place people turn when they lose a loved one due to a medication error. In fact, it is usually much later, when other avenues have been exhausted, that someone discovers a toll-free number for reporting side effects or medication errors or simply for questions about their medications.

This is where I work, at the other end of (888) INFO-FDA, in the U.S. Food and Drug Administration's Division of Drug Information, a division staffed by health care professionals who answer all inquiries including adverse event reporting to MEDWATCH. I work alongside other pharmacists and colleagues who take calls from patients experiencing the worst-case scenario when it comes to their medications. Every day and every call are different. In this job, you are not just a pharmacist, you are a source of kindness, understanding, and empathy to callers who have experienced an adverse event. Some callers want someone in the government to blame, and we listen. Other callers want someone to take the time to discuss their medications with them, and we talk. Many callers want someone to say, "I understand why you're upset," and to listen to their story, and we do. And then, there are callers who tell their story and elicit such a deep emotional reaction, you're not quite sure how they're on the other end of the line telling the story at all.

An example of the last type of call came from a woman who had recently lost her brother from a sudden cardiac arrest when he was younger than 40. Her brother had been prescribed varying doses of an atypical antipsychotic for off-label use and had been given a diagnosis of cardiomegaly; also, he had experienced almost 100 pounds of weight gain since beginning treatment for schizophrenia. He had a tumultuous medication history, with many different doses of the same medication. The month before his death, he filled a prescription for 100 mg daily and, at the first of the next month, filled a prescription for 600 mg daily. He died 2 days later from sudden cardiac arrest. The autopsy report stated that the cause of death was inappropriate medication use.

Listening to this woman report her brother's medical history and prescription record, while maintaining complete professional and emotional composure, was challenging. Probing for information on medical history, listening to her recount the erratic prescriptions her brother had been receiving, and hearing her concerns about his increasing weight were gut wrenching, as it seemed impersonal to ask the standard form questions but important to gather the full history nonetheless. Laboratory results and other questions like "Did he have any allergies?," "Did he have any kidney or liver problems?," and "Did he use tobacco or alcohol?" felt cold and insensitive to ask this woman, who was trying so hard to keep her emotions from spilling over.

Once the reporting process was finished, the woman broke down. She explained that her brother was her best friend, the closest person to her in the whole world, and that she has had to distance herself from the pain of losing him to be able to take action after his death. She thanked me for my time and assistance with the reporting process, and then we hung up. I was unprepared for how deeply moved I felt after speaking with this woman. After a few moments to regain my composure, it was time to answer the next call, and possibly be a shoulder for another person.

As pharmacists and members of the health care system, we take an oath to apply our knowledge, experience, and skills to the best of our ability to ensure optimal outcomes for our patients. What isn't mentioned in that oath is what to do when the system fails. We aren't taught how to empathetically address the loved ones of a patient who lost his life, and we aren't handed a script with compassionate words and phrases to comfort that person when she asks why this happened. What we do have is a quality inherent to human beings to be there for one another in a time of need, and it is this quality, along with our learned skills and experiences, that uniquely qualifies us as pharmacists to comfort our patients when all else fails.

Care from the Other Side of the Counter and Bedside

Pharmacists as Patients and Caregivers

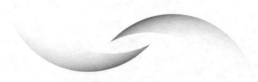

Could a greater miracle take place than for us to look through each other's eyes for an instant?

Henry David Thoreau

No man is a good doctor who has never been sick himself.

Chinese Proverb

Two Pharmacists

Katie S. McClendon, Pharm.D., BCPS
Educator

A Pharmacist Killed My Grandmother
Of course, it is not so simple. Things never are. A pharmacist made a mistake when two physicians were not aware of all the medications a patient was taking—a pretty common occurrence. The pharmacist dispensed high-dose sulfamethoxazole/trimethoprim to a 92-year-old woman taking warfarin but did not contact either of her physicians to notify them of the potential interaction. The pharmacist did not tell my grandmother or her daughter about the potential risk. My grandmother continued taking both medicines until one night she fell and broke her hip and had an INR so high that most labs would not bother to report the number.

A Pharmacist Restored My Faith in the Profession
Once my grandmother was hospitalized, I reached out to pharmacists I knew practicing near her hospital. I was able to talk with the pharmacist on my grandmother's team, and from 300 miles away, I was able to help communicate what was happening to the rest of my family. I have always appreciated the pharmacist taking the time to listen to me as well as to answer the many previously unanswered questions about what is happening in the hospital. Before talking to the pharmacist, sometimes I felt like I was playing a dangerous game of "telephone" with my grandmother's medical details, leaving me unable to help my family understand. My grandmother never recovered from the fall and hospitalization and died several months later.

Daughter of a Pharmacist
My grandmother's father was a pharmacist. He graduated from the Atlanta College of Pharmacy in 1904, 101 years before I graduated from pharmacy school. I now have his class composite hanging in my office, along with several other items reflecting his brief practice of pharmacy before he went back to school to become a physician. My

grandmother grew up not trusting medicine. According to my mother, my grandmother's father always told her that medicine was for "other people" since the most commonly prescribed medicine her father used was opium. I remember conversations with her when I was in pharmacy school and she was 90 years old. At that time, she took only once-weekly alendronate but detested the routine of taking medicine and then waiting around 30 minutes before having anything to eat or drink. As a resident, I often told this story to patients with a large and complicated medication regimen. I told them that it was a matter of your attitude; you could see medications as a burden, or you could just be grateful you didn't have it as bad as others did. One of my patients with diabetes and atrial fibrillation took more pills on a daily basis than my grandmother took in 3 months. But he loved the story of my grandmother and her one pill. Every time he came to see me, he asked how my grandmother was doing, always concerned about her osteoporosis. He passed away soon after my residency ended, and not much later, my grandmother was diagnosed with atrial fibrillation and a stroke. After this, she took a complex medication regimen which now included warfarin and amiodarone, a regimen rivaling that of my former patient, but her attitude toward medicine never changed much.

Grandmother of a Pharmacist
By the time my grandmother was placed on warfarin, I was a clinical pharmacist whose practice included an anticoagulation clinic. I regularly see the interaction that led to my grandmother's death, but thankfully, my patients have had much safer outcomes. I discuss it with students in problem-based learning discussions or on rotation. I teach each new warfarin patient (and any caregivers) to always remind every provider that they take warfarin and to ask, "Is this medicine OK to take with my warfarin?" This year, I wrote a case for students about my grandmother. I have yet to receive a long-distance call from a colleague asking me to check on a family member, but I would not hesitate to respond. I try to remind students that patients are not strangers. They are someone's grandmother. And I try to remind students that they can choose to be the pharmacist who may cause harm or the pharmacist who restores faith. I hope they choose well.

The Other Side of the Counter

Ashley Wimberly Ellis, Pharm.D.
Patient

On February 14, 2011, my beautiful baby girl arrived after months of planning, research, and anxious waiting. Along with her arrival came a flood of emotion that overwhelmed my heart and spirit. As a first-time mom, I felt intense joy, immense responsibility, and an intoxicating love unequal to any I had ever known. I was thrilled to bring my little bundle of joy into the world and into our home.

To ensure I took my pain medication on schedule, my hospital nurses suggested I leave my prescriptions at my pharmacy and let someone return for them after we settled in at home. Five cars slowly moving through the pharmacy drive-through lane and a crying newborn did not make a good combination. Ignoring my husband's advice, I got out of the car at the grocery entrance and hobbled to the pharmacy, after instructing him to drive around the parking lot to lull the baby to sleep. I handed my discharge orders to the pharmacist and asked him to put a large bottle of ibuprofen with my prescriptions. I had not kept ibuprofen in the house during my pregnancy because of the risks of taking it while pregnant. I explained to the pharmacist that my husband would pick up the prescriptions and ibuprofen at one time. As I turned to go, he told me where ibuprofen was located and said he would include it with my medicines if I brought it back to him before I left the store. I thought I had misunderstood him. It was just a few days after the birth of my first child and my surgery, I was clearly having trouble walking, and my prescriptions were written on hospital discharge papers stating why I was admitted and the need for each medication. I thought about discussing his attitude and customer service with him, but I needed to get back to my little family quickly. So I smoothed my ruffled feathers and slowly shuffled to the aisle he had indicated to search for the ibuprofen. The combination of pain medication–induced drowsiness, my difficulty walking, and the anxiety I felt at leaving my baby the first time for even a few minutes made this search seem much longer than it actually was. In spite of this, I found the ibuprofen and brought the bottle back to the pharmacist to include with my medications.

From a patient's perspective, I felt I did not receive the best possible care from this pharmacist. Had I been any other patient, with no training or knowledge of medications, who was sent to search for a medication that could make an enormous impact on a person's quality of life, pain, and ability to nurse a newborn baby—yet with the same physical limitations I was suffering after delivering a child—this task would have been much more difficult, if not impossible. Picking up a bottle from an over-the-counter shelf seems like a small task to the health care professional, but it is not such a small task to a person in pain. From the perspective of a pharmacist who has practiced in community pharmacy, I too have felt the compelling need to complete the immediate task at hand, whether stapling bags, scanning bar codes, answering the phone, or checking prescriptions for accuracy. I have also experienced the additional pressure of completing each of these tasks with absolute precision, efficiency, and accuracy. I know exactly how it feels to fill 300 prescriptions by noon without getting a lunch or bathroom break while giving flu shots between checking prescriptions. I also understand that a pharmacist's feelings of being overloaded can be compounded by a person who asks an apparently frivolous question. I too am guilty of thoughts like "I didn't spend all of those years in school to ring up someone's groceries!" or "If I had only one more technician today, I could go above and beyond what is required of a health care professional, but today, I can do only what is asked of me." If my thoughts and experience describe this pharmacist, I can understand a pharmacist having a bad day.

However, fast-forward 6 weeks to when my sweet baby girl and I celebrated my birthday by spending the day together. When I went to get her after an afternoon nap, I found a birthday surprise. Instead of seeing her precious smile, I saw the distressed frown of a crying baby. This was the cry that many of my experienced mom friends had talked about, but I never quite understood until I heard it myself. It was high-pitched and loud, and she was inconsolable. My usual tricks of rocking, playing, singing, and walking around failed miserably to soothe her. I had a sinking feeling something was wrong. After 1 hour, four diapers, and a call to the pediatrician's office, it was confirmed—she had her first stomach virus. Through my research before the baby arrived, I learned that stomach pains and gas are very painful for babies. My heart hurt for her to be that small, that helpless, and to feel that kind of pain for the first time. She couldn't possibly know what caused it, but she had no one but me to make everything better. Her crying tied my stomach in knots and made me want to cry, too. My pediatrician recommended simethicone drops, requiring a trip to the pharmacy. Surely, a ride in the car to get them would also make her feel better. No such luck! Her cries became louder and more frantic and made me more determined than ever to get her that medicine.

As I stopped at the drive-through of the very same pharmacy I had previously visited, I asked the same pharmacist for simethicone drops. He said he did not have time to help me with things like that. I was stunned! I could not believe my ears! My daughter's screaming and crying escalated, along with my anxiety level. I told him I was alone, with a screaming baby in the back seat, and asked him again for the medicine. Once again, he said he didn't have time to get the medicine. I immediately left and purchased the medicine at another pharmacy. She was comforted by the drops and recovered fully within a few days, but I learned a lesson I will never forget. A symptom as simple as gas pain in an infant became greatly magnified because the infant patient was my daughter. I wonder how many of my patients have been young, first-time mothers with babies, leaving the house for one of the first times in search of excellent health care at their pharmacy, but I failed to serve them to the best of my ability because I had not yet experienced the birth of my first child and all the love, worries, and special moments that came into my life when she did. Those mothers had a sick child just like mine. I should have helped a little more, shared a kind word or a smile, and even gone around to the other side of the counter to comfort them.

Those who are sick—babies, the elderly, middle-aged patients who have just been diagnosed with diabetes, and people who have a father, mother, or spouse in hospice care—are real people with real health crises. They walk into our community pharmacies every day and come face to face with a health care professional who has the opportunity to make life better, or at least a little more bearable, even if for only a few moments. We who serve as pharmacists can provide medications to make our patients feel better physically and can express sympathy and provide caring service to make them feel better emotionally and spiritually. Finding myself on the other side of the counter, I began to understand empathy. I know I will look at my 82-year-old patient whose diabetes I manage with a fresh appreciation for the obstacles and hurdles she experienced after the death of her husband. Her eating habits changed because her life, faith, and confidence had been shaken to its foundation after the loss of her best friend and companion. I know I will speak kinder words of encouragement to my 30-year-old patient with uncontrolled asthma symptoms caused by the smoking she picked up again after losing her job and being forced to move back home with her parents.

When the roles of pharmacist and patient were reversed, I realized the difference a pharmacist could make in the life of a scared, first-time mom with her emotions running in high gear. I learned that 5 minutes of my time could make a patient's next few hours and days a little more bearable. The role reversal inspired me to do more for my patients and reminded me that my profession is more than just placing pills in a bottle perfectly every time. It is serving people. Because of a new sense of empathy and a renewed understanding of my calling to pharmacy, a few more scared, emotional, first-time moms will get the medicine they need for their babies as easily as possible; will have one less worry of motherhood; and will experience compassionate care from a pharmacist.

You Give Them the Medicines and Make Them Feel Better

Katherine R. Fitz, Pharm.D.
PGY 2 Critical Care Pharmacy Resident

"What made you decide that you wanted to become a pharmacist?" It is one of my favorite questions to ask our residency candidates because you can never predict the answers you will hear. Some are inspired by family members, others have witnessed grotesque sights in the emergency department and decided pharmacy was easier to stomach, and still others have started as nurses' aides...but every pharmacist has a story to tell. I decided to become a pharmacist when I was 17 years old. I was a senior in high school and captain of the varsity swim team. I woke up at 4:45 a.m. and was in the pool by 5:30 a.m. It was not uncommon for me to swim more than 6 miles a day, and I was in excellent shape! With a challenging course load in addition to swim practices, I was busy, but things could not have been better.

Slowly, however, I started to notice that my body was becoming stiff in my hands, feet, and knees. I attributed it to the cold November weather in Michigan and to running around with wet hair after practice...or maybe it was caused by the hundreds of flip-turns that I did on a daily basis. Never the type of person to turn to the doctor with the slightest discomfort, I waited to feel better, but relief never came. Instead, the pain worsened until it became so bad that I would sit on my bathroom counter to get ready for school in the mornings to avoid enduring the pain of standing on my feet. The ring that I had inherited from my grandma no longer fit over my swollen fingers. I had promised my mom after a round of hepatitis vaccines I had received as a 12-year-old, "When I'm 18, I'm never going to the doctor again." How plans change.

After Lamaze-breathing my way through a blood draw, my diagnosis was made: I had rheumatoid arthritis. I was not sure what to think. I had never taken a prescription before, and Celebrex was a drug that my friend's dad took for a tennis injury. I had no comprehension of the severity of my disease until I had failed a few rounds of different medications with no symptom relief. My hands were so swollen and stiff that I was unable to curl my fingers enough to open my prescription bottles. It was then that my rheumatologist started me on etanercept injections and methotrexate. What a regimen for a 17-year-old to understand! I had not been to the doctor since the hepatitis vaccines, and I had not experienced a blood draw until the time of my diagnosis. I was told that I would be starting every-other-Monday blood draws, injecting myself twice a week, taking methotrexate on Wednesdays, taking Celebrex twice daily. I tried to clarify this regimen several times, and it was a lot to take in. I insisted that under no circumstances would I be able to inject myself! I planned to make the 1-hour round trip drive twice a week to the hospital for the injections.

I had never felt so hopeless. Always the optimist, I felt, for once, that I had nothing to be optimistic about. For all of my exercise and healthy eating habits, I was completely blindsided by this diagnosis. My dad cried on the drive to the hospital, saying, "I don't know why this had to happen to you, Katherine. You are such a good person!" What was worse was that I knew that I would live with this disease for the rest of my life. For a 17-year-old, that is an especially long time.

With a natural aptitude for math and science, I had planned to become an engineer like my dad. My mom, a nursing administrator, tried to persuade me into pharmacy: "Pharmacists are some of the smartest people I know! You would be such a good pharmacist!" she always said. In a situation where I felt as though I had lost all control, I realized that pharmacy would be a way in which I could regain it. I felt that if I acquired a better understanding of my disease and the medications, it would be easier for me to accept. In the last semester of my senior year of high school, I shadowed a pharmacist, and I was hooked. My family and I shared more tears, although this time, they were joyful ones when we learned of my acceptance into the Early Admissions Pathway program at The Ohio State University. I remember the exact moment and where we were standing when we found out. That moment changed my life.

The more I learned about the profession, the more I idolized pharmacists. I worked as a technician at a hospital, and although the manager warned me that it "wasn't a glamour job," I loved being part of the inpatient pharmacy. Most of my daily responsibility revolved around preparing and delivering medications to the nursing units. As I pushed a cart carrying almost 20 liters of continuous bladder irrigation solution through the hallway, I realized what my manager meant when he made the comment about the lack of glamour. I was interested in learning about the medications, though, and I credit most of my knowledge of brand/generic drug names to that job. It was surprising how much I was able to learn about the daily operations of a hospital pharmacy, the commonly used medications, and pharmacist participation in medical emergencies. Recognizing my passion for the profession, the pharmacists made an extra effort to explain various therapeutic concepts to me as I listened in awe. The student organizations at Ohio State often invited pharmacists to speak to us about their careers. During these lunch sessions, I was so inspired! The pharmacists would casually mention how they would catch drug interactions and duplications in therapy or how they would make recommendations for optimizing the patient's current regimens. To me, pharmacists were like superheroes! I only hoped to one day be half as clever.

After my first year of college, my arthritis was under much better control, and I knew I was lucky to have responded so well to treatment. Despite the hundreds of injections I had given myself since my diagnosis, my fear of needles never dissipated, and I still had to psyche myself up by listening to music to do the injections. I would set deadlines that I could never meet: "1, 2, 3...OK, this time I really will do this...1, 2, 3... nope...." On bad days, I would sit shaking, holding the needle above my skin and crying while trying to coax my fears away long enough just to get the dreaded injection over with. My rheumatologist inspired me with this quote from Thucydides: "But the palm of courage will surely be adjudged most justly to those, who best know the difference between hardship and pleasure and yet are never tempted to shrink from danger." Despite the bad injection days, things were much better overall, and I had returned to my optimistic self.

During my third year of pharmacy school, my dad had a hemicolectomy to remove a suspicious mass. Thankfully, the mass turned out to be benign, but my dad's recovery was complicated. The day before Thanksgiving, he was suffering from tremendous pain in his lower back. My mom called the physician, who thought it sounded like a urinary tract infection. He was ready to write a prescription for antibiotics, but my mom, a nurse, insisted that it was not a UTI. She saved his life. My dad was brought in for a CT scan, which revealed a clot in his superior mesenteric vein. He was started on enoxaparin injections and warfarin. My mom and I spent the week in tears after learning that the associated mortality from this type of clot is about 30 percent. Although I was not engaged, we wondered about my wedding without my dad to walk me down the aisle. It was a very stressful time, but my dad's clot slowly disappeared. It was then that I became interested in anticoagulation. To my dad, protein C deficiency seemed to be a sign that his body was wearing out. Otherwise healthy, he hated the idea of taking a prescription and the blood draws that it required. I explained to him that the coagulopathy had always been present and was not a sign of aging. During the past few years, I have answered more than a few dozen warfarin-related questions for him. Acceptance comes through knowledge of one's disease and its treatment. I am fortunate to have the opportunity to be that resource for my dad.

In 2010, I graduated from pharmacy school. It was such a special day! I thought back to when I was 17 and the promise I had made to myself to take control over my disease. Not only had I learned how to be my own advocate, but I had also been able to help my dad through his blood clot and answer dozens of warfarin-related questions for him. Although physicians make the diagnosis and determine what is wrong with a patient, pharmacists have the opportunity to make it right. What a sense of power I have found in that knowledge! Pharmacy is such a unique and honorable profession, and I cannot think of any title I would be prouder to be called than "Pharmacist." No matter the tone of the person on the other end of the phone, I always feel a surge of pride when I say, "Yes, I am a pharmacist."

Currently, I am completing a critical care residency at a large teaching hospital. I am pursuing a teaching certificate so that I can be a more effective preceptor, and I am actively involved in research. In my first year as a pharmacist, I submitted one of my studies, which evaluated the use of a warfarin-dosing nomogram, for publication. Through these educational efforts to improve anticoagulation outcomes at my institution, the frequency of pharmacy consultation for warfarin management has doubled. My mom's coworker mentioned that she ran into me at the hospital. "She seemed really happy," she told her of our encounter. I *am* really happy. Through my hardship, I have discovered my true passion. Rheumatoid arthritis, blood clots…: these diseases do not sound as dramatic as cancer or some of the medical conditions portrayed on television; but for the patient, these diagnoses are life-changing. As pharmacists, we have an incredible opportunity to educate patients, nurses, physicians, and family members. Through this education, we can help alleviate fears and empower patients to take control over their diagnoses. We teach patients how to use medications properly, soothe them as we provide immunizations, and decode the foreign language of medical-speak. Behind the scenes, we optimize therapeutic regimens, monitoring for drug interactions, adverse events, and efficacy. For these opportunities to affect patient care, I am grateful. Reflecting on my personal struggle, I hope to improve the care of others.

As I was walking through the hospital the other day, I smiled at a small child. He smiled back at me in my white coat and asked, "Are you a doctor?" For simplicity's sake, I said "yes," to which he replied: "And you give them the medicines and make them feel better?" I smiled and nodded.

Lessons My Mother Taught Me

Shannon H. Goldwater, Pharm.D., FASHP, BCPS
Clinician/Educator/Preceptor

Throughout my 31-year pharmacy career, my mother has been there to help shape me into the pharmacist I am today. She patiently reviewed the top 200 drugs, even though she could hardly pronounce drug names. As an educator, she helped me appreciate that education is a gift, one that I should continue to craft. My two pharmacy degrees armed me with many critical tools to assist me as a pharmacist. But for me, the most meaningful lessons are those that my mother has taught me in the past 5 years as one of her direct caregivers. She has embodied for me what Hilton Head, San Antonio, and now the recent Pharmacy Practice Model Summit[1] are directing that we, as pharmacists, should be doing—providing patient drug information, tailoring drug therapy to fit the patient's lifestyle, instilling patient confidence, and proactively applying evidence-based guidelines to prevent and/or limit disease.

Surprisingly, my mother has had very few encounters with health care throughout her 89 years, despite smoking cigarettes for close to 65 years. But eventually, she suffered the consequences of smoking: abdominal aortic aneurysm (AAA), stroke, myocardial infarction, CABG, and oxygen-dependent chronic obstructive pulmonary disease. From her perspective, she went into the hospital "healthy" and came out a train wreck.

After a lengthy hospital and skilled nursing facility stay, Mom transitioned home. As I stepped into my new caregiver role for my mother, I began to see health care from an entirely different perspective—that of the chronic care patient. As you can imagine, my mother's drug regimen included numerous drugs using several different modes of delivery, all of which were new for her. I took a traditional pharmacy role: I provided drug information. As I observed her technique with her respiratory medications, it was clear that she needed to be taught how and when to use these medications. Over the course of my career, hospital pharmacy had left most of the medication teaching to nursing, and with the few medications for which we did provide direct patient teaching, we complained about how much time it took!

It was easy to see that with 18 different medications, Mom was having difficulty figuring out what to take and when to take it. A medication calendar helped her see the pills through all the pill bottles. After I interviewed my mom to learn of her daily habits, we determined together the optimal time to take her medicines that fit into her routine, rather than change her life to fit around taking medicine, which she was most definitely fighting. We even eliminated a few medications that often remain after an intensive care stay: goodbye, proton pump inhibitor! Mom is now equipped with a simpler drug regimen that works around her, not the other way around. However, this has not been enough.

It became apparent after her hospital and nursing facility stay that Mom lacked confidence in her ability to perform this task of daily medication-taking consistently. My mother often worries about her memory. Yet it is difficult to recall whether a task is completed when it is interrupted by a phone call. For that, it has been satisfying to see that using weekly pillboxes for Mom's medicines has greatly improved her confidence in her pill-taking behaviors. If you are a pharmacist, you should not be surprised at any of the steps I have taken to provide care for my mother; after all, they are "pharmacy-centric" tasks, which is what we were taught to do in pharmacy school. Sad to say, though, it seems like only pharmacy students perform these functions on a regular basis. But Mom reminds me of the importance of these tasks even as she improves on her ability to accurately and consistently carry out her medication-taking behaviors.

During this journey of caring for my mother, I have obtained board certification in pharmacotherapy. As expected, obtaining my BCPS has enhanced my knowledge base and filled in gaps of new areas of drug development. What I did not expect was a newfound confidence in my abilities.

With this renewed knowledge base and newfound confidence, I have received numerous opportunities to be proactive in my mother's care, and ways that could make a tremendous difference in her quality of life have leapt in front of my eyes. These opportunities to be proactive are the very things that are integral to health care reform. Information and incentives are two major barriers to consistently delivering high-quality care that are addressed by the Affordable Care

Act.[2] Removing these barriers is likely to result in preventive care, finding ways to reduce hospital readmissions, and engaging patients in health care decisions. The patient-centered medical home (PCMH) is a team, including pharmacists, that functions as the focal point of patient information, primary care provision, and care coordination. The PCMH team facilitates the delivery of evidence-based disease management and patient self-management services.[3] Health care is forced to shift to a proactive stance when the goal is to prevent disease and/or identify disease earlier in a patient-centric environment in which the patient assumes responsibility for his/her health and wellness. The American College of Clinical Pharmacy's position paper on Healthy People 2010 identifies several key roles for pharmacy.[4] Clinical preventive care and primary care are among the many vital duties for pharmacy as we move toward Healthy People 2020, particularly as it pertains to counseling about health behaviors such as diet, exercise, smoking cessation, or drug management. Pharmacy needs to document its efforts as we provide a growing public health function. Looking back to before I obtained board certification, what were some of the missed opportunities in which I, as a pharmacist, could have facilitated better care for my mother?

The NCEP/ATP guidelines[5] identify smoking, hypertension, low HDL, family history of premature coronary heart disease (CHD), age, diabetes, peripheral arterial disease, AAA, and symptomatic carotid artery disease as CHD or CHD risk equivalents. Patients with CHD or CHD risk equivalents should be treated with a statin to an LDL goal of less than 100 mg/dL. Given my mother's history of AAA, she should have received a statin when her AAA was identified to prevent cardiovascular disease, especially given her smoking history. Unfortunately, this addition came after her myocardial infarction, so secondary prevention is now the goal.

Advanced age, female sex, menopause, and a fracture often indicate the presence of osteoporosis.[6] Known modifiable risk factors for osteoporosis include smoking, low-calcium diet, heavy alcohol use, inactive lifestyle, and certain medication use. My mother has had three fractures since she was 60. However, it was not until she was given the diagnosis of a spinal compression fracture at age 88 that a bisphosphonate was added to her regimen.

The 2008 update of U.S. Department of Health and Human Services' Treating Tobacco Use and Dependence[7] identified that smokers see several health care providers every year, including pharmacists. A 3-minute intervention can have a substantial impact on motivating smokers to quit. However, many health care providers find talking with a smoker either frustrating or too sensitive. I will admit that, as my mother's child, I took the baseball bat approach and beat her up about the risks of smoking, which was very ineffective. But in the past few years, I have found that motivational interviewing is an effective way to reach patients, including my mother, who are resistant to change.[8]

As I reflect on my 31-year career, I value what my mother has taught me through the years—and what she continues to teach me. At the center of every decision in health care is a patient: a person with a name, a face, and a family that cares about the patient's existence. If I could change one thing about my career path, it would be to have understood the patient perspective earlier in my career. This would have allowed me to be a better advocate for the hospital and pharmacy programs that benefit the patients we serve. The impact of this perspective on my career has helped me ensure that each pharmacy student gains this perspective during his or her rotation with me. I often use aspects of my mother's care to help pharmacy students appreciate the patient perspective. Then, I encourage students to talk with their family members to help them gain this insight, as it is easier for them to talk with a family member than for them to ask more probing questions.

Learning to view health care from the 20,000-foot level, to gain the perspective of the potential of our profession and of me as an individual, has been very informative. Even more enlightening has been gaining that patient perspective to humanize the very essence of what I wanted to do with pharmacy in the first place. As I stand on the threshold of change for pharmacy, I am even more excited to see the tremendous opportunities that exist for me today to do more in caring for patients who need our help. Through the years, Mom has encouraged my siblings and me to be actively engaged rather than content to do the minimum to keep our jobs. For me, I strive to find better ways of providing health care. Although I cannot always say that I have loved every minute of every job I have ever held, I can say that I more fully appreciate the patient experience of health care because of my mother. As a result, I am happy, satisfied, and excited to have done what I have and continue to do. Thanks, Mom, for helping me learn to be a better health care provider. I hope my students and my readers have also learned at your bedside.

My mother recently passed away. Even while dying, she had one final lesson to teach. The ultimate in patient care is realizing that medicine cannot always alter the outcome. We have to possess the wisdom to recognize the moment and the courage to respect the patient's wish to simply die with dignity.

1. Pharmacy Practice Model Summit. Executive summary. Am J Health Syst Pharm 2011; 68:e43–4.
2. Kocher R, Emanuel EJ, DeParle NAM. The Affordable Care Act and the future of clinical medicine: The opportunities and challenges. Ann Intern Med 2010;153:536–9.
3. American College of Physicians. Policy Paper. The Patient-Centered Medical Home Neighbor: The Interface of the Patient-Centered Medical Home with Specialty/Subspecialty Practices. Philadelphia: American College of Physicians, 2010.
4. Calis KA, Hutchison LC, Elliott ME, et al. Healthy People 2010: Challenges, opportunities, and a call to action for America's pharmacists. Pharmacotherapy 2004;24:1241–94.
5. Expert Panel on Detection, Evaluation, and Treatment of High Blood Cholesterol in Adults. Executive summary of the third report of the National Cholesterol Education Program (NCEP). JAMA 2001;285:2486–97.
6. Qaseem A, Snow V, Shekelle P, et al. Pharmacologic treatment of low bone density or osteoporosis to prevent fractures: A clinical practice guideline from the American College of Physicians. Ann Intern Med 2008;149:404–15.
7. Fiore MC, Jaen CR, Baker TB, et al. Treating Tobacco Use and Dependence: 2008 Update. Clinical Practice Guideline. Rockville, Md.: U.S. Department of Health and Human Services, Public Health Service, May 2008.
8. Scales R, Miller J, Burden R. Why wrestle when you can dance? Optimizing outcomes with motivational interviewing. J Am Pharm Assoc 2003;43(5 Suppl 1):S46–S47.

Both Sides of the Bedside

Kayla E. Smith, Pharm.D.
Student

A s a pharmacy student and future health care professional, I've always wanted to help people. In fact, I have been told to treat every patient as if he or she were one of my own grandparents. Ironically, during my first clinical rotation this summer, I happened to be at the hospital where my *mémère* (grandmother) was admitted as a patient. My experience shuffling from pharmacy student back to granddaughter taught me a lot about our health care system, the people involved in it, and the power of patient advocates.

At the teaching hospital, the medical residents often consulted me when medication-related questions arose about their patients. While rounding with the medical team in my first rotation, I was able to meet many patients, some frustrated with being in the hospital. I tried to empathize with them, knowing that our team was trying to help make them better. I was able to see how hard the young physicians worked to care for their patients and how much they cared. Being on the health care side of the situation made me realize why it took so long to change a medication dose, take a patient for a simple CT scan, or discharge a patient from the hospital. The effort put forth every day by the health care team was impressive, commendable, and selfless.

When my *mémère* was admitted, our family was very concerned about the amount of pain she was in and about the cause. My *mémère*, we knew, had metastatic breast cancer, and we were worried about what this pain meant. The pain medication originally prescribed was not working at all. After she had been almost 12 hours with 10/10 on the pain scale, I asked her doctor if we could try a different agent. However, he wanted to wait a little longer. After 18 agonizing hours, I asked a different doctor, who agreed to prescribe something different. Her relief was instant—our relief followed. The pain problem was solved for the time being. As a pharmacy student, I knew how easily mistakes could occur in the health care system. Before I left for the evening, I checked with the nurse to be sure her original pain medication would be stopped. She assured me that it would. The next morning, I arrived to find my grandmother extremely drowsy. The night nurse wanted to stop giving the pain medication that was working because he felt it was too much for her. Looking at her, I agreed, but I explained how the original medication did not seem to help her pain. They finally agreed to leave her on the stronger agent. Had I not been there to speak up, my grandmother would have been put back on the original medication that was not working. Later that night, we found out that she had been receiving both medications during the nightshift, despite my efforts to ensure this didn't happen, and that the excess sedation was, in fact, from the dual therapy. Without my insistence, she would have been continued on the medication that wasn't helping her pain because of a communication error that could have been prevented. It was a breakdown in the system.

This is just one instance of the system-related problems that occurred. In the following few days, she had three CT scans, one x-ray, two endoscopies, and one echocardiogram, yet still, no one had any answers for what was causing the pain. Some days, no one told the family why these tests were even being done. After learning she was having an esophageal bleed, I had to intervene when a nurse was about to administer her scheduled anticoagulant. The order had not yet been written to discontinue it because the doctors on her team had not yet been told the results of the endoscopy that ultimately revealed the bleed. This was not the last time I had to speak up regarding her care. Upon discharge, there were a few interventions with missing prescriptions and correcting instructions. Acting only as her granddaughter, I always respected the boundaries of her protected health information.

The system has so much room for error. It is not necessarily a people problem, but rather, a system problem. What has this experience taught me about our health care system and my future role as a pharmacist? It has increased my awareness of how many opportunities there are for errors within the health care system. The entire health care team has a responsibility to look for where errors can occur and be vigilant in closing those gaps. This experience has made me more attentive to the needs of the patients and their families: to ask if they have any questions, to listen to their concerns, and to communicate with them about their health care. It has also taught me about the importance of patient advocates, whether a family member, the patient themselves, or a member of the health care staff. I encourage all pharmacy students and residents, as well as current health care professionals, to be aware of the needs and concerns of patients and their families because someday you may find yourself on the other side of the bedside.

Acknowledgment:
I would like to acknowledge and thank Anne Hume, Pharm.D., for her guidance and support during this experience.

Dire Situations

Care amid Catastrophe

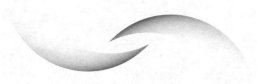

*Nothing has more strength than
dire necessity.*

Euripides

*Wherever a man turns he can find
someone who needs him.*

Albert Schweitzer

Letting the Mission Define Your Role: Reflections from the Battlefield

Felix K. Yam, Pharm.D.
Chief Pharmacy Officer

S hamrock Black, Shamrock Black, Shamrock Black. That call sign echoes in my ears 2 years after my 12-month tour as a military pharmacist attached to a combat unit deployed to a remote region of Afghanistan.

This call sign was blasted through the forward operating base loudspeakers to alert the surgical team and any other available soldiers of incoming casualties from the battlefield when insurgents, attempting to enter our base disguised, together with other local workers from neighboring villages, failed to breach the perimeter but managed to detonate themselves before they could be disarmed. "Shamrock Black" meant that we had a mass casualty event with numbers injured instantly exceeding our forward surgical team's capabilities and requiring an "all-hands-on-deck" approach as soldiers, from supply technicians to engineers, would jump in to answer the call. Within minutes, our trauma teams, along with other soldiers, would converge on the makeshift field hospital to prepare for receiving the most critical casualties.

Our surgical team consisted of a general surgeon, an orthopedic surgeon, a nurse anesthetist, a trauma nurse, a medic, an operating room technician, a pharmacy technician, and a pharmacist. Our mission was simple, to protect each other and save lives. To do this, we were all trained as combat medics, whose primary focus was to find the source of the bleed, stop the bleed, prepare the soldier for return to duty, or prepare the soldier for transfer to the next level of care. On the worst days, the mission was to prepare the soldier for travel back to the United States draped with an American flag. To accomplish our mission, we were all prepared to do each other's jobs. Under these circumstances, our technical roles or job titles did not define who we were; rather, we let the mission define our roles.

As I reflect on these experiences, I realize how important it is to understand that a mission can unite soldiers and people alike to function as a team and work as one unit. During my tour, I learned the true meaning of selfless service, sacrifice, and professionalism. I am not referring to my own service and sacrifice but to that of those whom I cared for, who seemingly gave so much more. As a health care professional and, more importantly, a fellow soldier, I owed them my best effort. Being a professional meant that I could not let my personal desires compromise the mission. I had to understand the importance of working with the team, united with a common purpose. There was no time for inflated egos or hesitation in performing tasks we were not fully trained to perform. Non–medically trained soldiers performed lifesaving combat first aid, nurses assisted with critical triaging services, pharmacists performed basic and advanced cardiac life support, pharmacy technicians started intravenous lines, and general surgeons performed miraculous procedures on a daily basis. No matter the task, time was of the essence, and we took action. Accomplishing the mission was so ingrained in our spirits that it became an obsession. Failure was not an option.

During mass casualty events, we all had to be technically proficient in our own roles, but more importantly, we had to have a deep sense of personal responsibility for the mission. Belief in the mission led soldiers to do extraordinary things. Heroes are made in this manner. On the day of one suicide bombing, our forward surgical team of 20 personnel cared for 56 casualties and achieved a 100 percent survival rate. This could not have been accomplished without the help of soldiers who refused to let their individual roles define them. Instead, they let the mission guide the actions they would perform that day. Their mission was simple—protect each other and save lives—and that is exactly they did.

In the hospital, I have sometimes heard a colleague proclaiming, "It's not my job" or "I am not trained"; such words are said to avoid doing a particular task. As I reflect on my deployment experience, I can think of several occasions when soldiers could have used those lines, but they didn't; it simply wasn't an option. Since my deployment, I have noticed myself reverting to the individual mind-set in which tasks and job duties are reduced to boxes to be checked off when completed; the shorter the list, the better the day. My sense of the mission is diluted just trying to keep up with the daily grind of pharmacy practice and the regulatory scrutiny that accompanies it. I have to consistently remind myself to see the bigger picture and understand how my role and daily actions contribute to the mission of my profession. If my mission is to improve the health of the patients I serve, then I should seek to overcome the barriers that prevent me from succeeding, much like the soldier who refuses to fail in the face of uncertainty and danger.

Although I understand that combat situations may not accurately represent the challenges pharmacists face in the civilian world, they teach us about the importance of understanding our mission as pharmacists and health care providers. The fundamental mission of all health professionals is the same, regardless of discipline or specialty. We are all servants of the public, seeking to improve others' health and to prolong the maximum quality of life. Pharmacists achieve this mission through promoting the best use of medications. Other professions achieve this mission through different means, but one thing is common: this mission unites all health care providers to serve a common purpose, similar to soldiers who are motivated by caring for their fellow brother or sister in arms. Regardless of the skill or trade held by individual soldiers, they let the mission guide their actions. As pharmacists, we, too, are guided by caring for the patients we serve and our colleagues who contribute to that effort.

Yet in practice, pharmacists have a tendency to build walls around their identity and create roles in which they can become very protective of what they do. For example, in the hospital under the same department, pharmacists specialize in drug distribution, sterile compounding, clinical service, drug information, investigational drugs, information technology, and many other areas. Each of these roles has a unique focus, and it is easy to move further away from the fundamentals of our training as we progress in them. Over time, we become very comfortable in these roles and allow them to limit our ability to contribute to the mission in other ways when necessary. Moreover, through the years, the health care industry has become highly regulated, and under this regulatory scrutiny, pharmacists have developed clearly defined roles requiring competency checklists, certification exams, and a litany of other educational requirements to perform daily tasks. In many ways, we have become so driven by policies and procedures that it is difficult to perform our jobs without them. Where procedures do not exist, we create them, and where policies do not exist, we establish them. In doing so, we have a tendency to confine ourselves to performing only the functions that are defined. In many ways, we have let our roles be defined by policies and procedures rather than shaped by the overarching mission of patient care.

My experience in Afghanistan, however, has made me realize that role definitions can sometimes build artificial barriers if we fail to adapt and be as flexible as the mission dictates. Knowing when to break down these barriers to accomplish the mission is critical. In a profession as diverse as pharmacy, it can be easy to forget that our fundamental training is the same, regardless of the roles that define us. More than ever before, we are in need of pharmacist leaders who can inspire others to take responsibility for achieving our profession's mission. I can remember my former pharmacy director at the University of Kentucky, who routinely beat his "Best Practice" drum as he walked the wards, as he passed you in the hallway, and as every department meeting began and ended. He took personal responsibility for achieving the mission and inspired his employees to do the same. Effective teams have a clear mission that is communicated often until it is deeply rooted in the spirit of all employees—pharmacy and otherwise.

Reflections from a Haitian Level One Trauma Center

Nicole J. Harger, Pharm.D., BCPS
Clinician

"And this is the pharmacy..." I tuned out the physician giving our tour as I looked around the exquisitely small pharmacy that I would be staffing the next week as part of a group medical mission trip to Port-au-Prince, Haiti. The door to the outside was wide open with no evidence of a lock or alarm. Multiple labeled bags hung on the wall by the door, all containing many syringes of different strengths of morphine. Wire carts filled with haphazard bins of medications sat in rows, taking up most of the space in the pharmacy. The IV compounding area consisted of an old medication cart sitting in the corner, mostly covered with opened vials and labeled syringes to be reused. I spied a small ant scurrying along the side of a Dextrose bag that was hanging for use as a diluent. The anal-retentive rule follower in me cringed inwardly, as I quickly reminded myself that I was in a Third World country that was recovering from a major natural disaster.

My shift wasn't scheduled to start until about an hour after the conclusion of our tour, so I wandered over to the emergency department (ED). There were no patients in the ED at the time, and I was quickly greeted with huge smiles from my nurse, physician, and respiratory care colleagues along with jovial teasing about already missing my presence with them in the ED. As I examined the two-bed department, my colleagues were quick to point out the boxes of random medications scattered throughout the room. We giggled about the vials and syringes of fentanyl and hydromorphone that were sitting out on the counters. I was glad that I was not the only person to find this lack of narcotic security so out of the ordinary, but I was also a little morose that they were all still able to work together and kid around while I would be by myself in the pharmacy.

I spent my first day in the pharmacy trying to become functional as quickly as possible. Training and figuring out the processes were challenging; I didn't speak much French Creole, and the Haitian pharmacist and technicians that I worked with didn't speak much English. We easily adapted a system of pointing and signing that made us laugh but allowed us to communicate more efficiently. I spent my downtime the first day sorting through the racks of medications to familiarize myself with what was available. I was amazed by the new and exciting medications that I found on the shelves as well as the sheer number of different drugs they had available. I also found some medications/medication classes to be notably absent from the shelves, a product of being mostly dependent on donations for pharmacy inventory.

One of the biggest units at the hospital was the pediatric unit. I work in an adult hospital with a children's hospital a block away, so my experience with pediatric medication information and dosing was extremely limited. Beginning on the first day, the one pediatric attending physician that accompanied us on our trip came to the pharmacy often, asking medication selection and pediatric dosing questions, looking more and more frazzled with each visit. After having a mini-MI while trying to look up the first pediatric dosing question, I began to assure myself that my limited pediatric drug knowledge was better than nothing, so we would have to make do.

The second day of our trip, I was becoming much more comfortable and familiar with the pharmacy. My Haitian technician and I took an instant liking to one another and had a great day together. It was almost the end of my 12-hour shift when the pediatric attending came flying through the door. "We have a new preemie with no prenatal care whose mother has confirmed HIV. We need to start antiretroviral therapy as soon as possible. Please figure out what he needs," she stated breathlessly as she ran back out the door. Luckily, I had spent a significant amount of time in our HIV clinic during my residency, so I was familiar with the proper treatment recommendations; I just needed to figure out the dosing. As I searched for dosing information for antiretroviral therapy in a 3-day-old preemie, I asked my technician if we had the medication available. We did not, so I moved on to the second-line therapy recommendations. We did have these available, but only in tablets. I calculated and recalculated the dose and decided that, without any kind of compounding vehicles, we would have to crush up the tablets and dilute them with water. After crushing the tablets, diluting them out, checking my math again, and drawing up the correct dose,

I ran the medications to the peds unit. As I walked in, I saw a look of relief on the attending's face. After reviewing the math and dosing with her, we explained everything to the nurse taking care of the patient, as well as to the patient's grandmother, who was sitting with him.

I was in awe at the number of family members present in the pediatric unit. Each child had at least one person accompanying them; many had two to four parents or grandparents with them. The family members took a very active role in the care of the patients. They fed them, bathed them, and sat quietly, reassuring the frightened and often fussy babies and children. As I would later discover, they also stayed overnight, sleeping on the tile floor of the pediatric unit or on the concrete benches in the courtyard.

Later in the week, the pediatric unit received a 2-year-old girl with hydrocephalus who was experiencing uncontrolled seizures. We worked diligently trying different therapies to break her seizures, with no success. The decision was finally made to intubate the patient and hook her up to the one very rudimentary ventilator that the hospital had. The medical director informed us in no uncertain terms that the rule for intubation in the pediatric unit at the hospital was that the patients had 24 hours on the ventilator; if they could not "fly" on their own after that, they would not be put back on ventilator. Although we understood that this rule was necessary to manage resources, it was a shocking prospect. I calculated the doses and drew up the intubation medications while the respiratory therapists tried to figure out the ventilator and the patient's mother bagged her. As I calculated the doses, I realized that the girl was drastically underweight, weighing in at just over 10 pounds.

After the girl was successfully intubated, we decided to give her phenobarbital. As I hastily grabbed her dose out of the (unlocked) narcotic drawer in the pharmacy, I realized that we had very few doses of phenobarbital left, as we had treated another seizing child the day before. I asked the technician to check for more stock in the cabinet, which was little more than a large portable shed with a padlock on it.

To the delight of the whole staff, the girl responded to the phenobarbital and stopped seizing. I returned to the pharmacy, eager to share the great news with my technician. She, however, had not so great news for me. We didn't have any phenobarbital in the overstock area. I immediately contacted the medical director to see if she would authorize an emergency trip to the warehouse to replenish our phenobarbital stock. A trip to the warehouse was arranged as we tried to ration the remaining phenobarbital while keeping the girl seizure free.

About 3 hours later, the supply manager came to the pharmacy with more unpleasant news. There was no phenobarbital in the warehouse. The medical director, along with one of our neurology attendings, the nurse manager, and I, met to figure out our options. The nurse manager began calling local hospitals to see if they could spare phenobarbital in exchange for a medication or supply that they needed. She finally found a hospital about 45 minutes away that was willing to trade us for our needed phenobarbital. We figured out that we had enough phenobarbital to last through the night; a trip to the other hospital was arranged for early the next day.

The next morning, shortly after I arrived for my 7:00 shift, the nurse manager came in to let me know that the supply manager was back from his trip to the other hospital, and she had more unpleasant news. Apparently, there was a misunderstanding; the other hospital had Purell hand sanitizer waiting for us instead of phenobarbital. We were coming very close to depleting our current stock and were quickly running out of options to replenish it. As I worked with the pediatric attending to brainstorm about any available medications that we hadn't tried and that might work as an alternative, we both realized that it was coming close to the 24-hour mark for the girl and her ventilator.

Precisely 24 hours after she was intubated, we extubated the little girl. It was quickly evident to everyone that she was not going to "fly" without the respiratory support. As we weaned her from the little phenobarbital we had left, she began seizing again. We tried alternative agents, but nothing seemed to work. After a discussion with her family, the decision was made to give her comfort care. I was in disbelief as I worked to calculate doses for medications to keep her comfortable; we definitely didn't learn about comfort care for children in school or residency!

I periodically took doses of morphine over to the pediatric unit and occasionally stayed to hold the girl's tiny hand or just watch her little body struggle to breathe. Finally, when it was apparent that the end was near, her mother held her as we all said our goodbyes. Her mother asked us to take a picture of them on her cell phone, which we did with tears in our eyes. As the little girl took her last breath, her mother was very stoic; the American staff was much more visibly upset, knowing that if this child had been born in different circumstances, the ending to her story would have likely been much happier.

Before we all went back to our duties, we reflected about how powerless we felt without the resources we were accustomed to and what a tragedy this huge discrepancy in the quality of health care resources was. We were well aware that the hospital we were staffing was the premiere hospital in Haiti, where people traveled miles and miles to be seen. It was hard to imagine the obstacles that the more rural hospitals were up against. Before leaving for our trip, we had received educational information about health care in Haiti as well as what to expect. We had learned many shocking statistics, such as that the average dollars per capita spent on health care in Haiti was around $83 (compared with $5,274 in the United States) and that one of every five children would die from malnutrition, dehydration, or diarrhea. While in Haiti, we were told that 1% of the Haitian people own 50% of the wealth in the country and that corruption prevented most of the aid money and supplies sent from overseas from ever reaching the people of Haiti. Although all of this information was both appalling and depressing, it didn't totally sink in until we experienced it ourselves. We felt powerless but reminded ourselves that each patient we helped and every health care professional we taught let us leave the health care situation in Haiti a little better than we found it.

We ended the conversation realizing that the girl was in a much better place, and no longer seizing. To this day, when I take care of seizing patients with any of my colleagues who went to Haiti, we always share a quick smile, knowing that we are both thinking of the girl seizure free and happy.

Pharmacy Response in Natural Disasters: Reflections from Hurricane Gustav

Amber Holdiness, Pharm.D.
Student

Kristen Pate, Pharm.D.
Student

Adam Pate, Pharm.D.
Student

Deborah S. Minor, Pharm.D.
Preceptor/Educator

After Hurricane Katrina destroyed the Gulf Coast in 2005, we were challenged with serving the medical needs of a large group of evacuees at a large shelter near the University of Mississippi Medical Center (UMMC) campus in Jackson. We learned from this experience and then used these lessons as we prepared for the ravages of Hurricane Gustav, almost exactly 3 years later.

As Hurricane Gustav was bearing down on the Louisiana–Mississippi Gulf Coast, volunteers at UMMC were poised to take action. Compared with our Katrina response, we were better prepared initially to meet the needs of our evacuee population. By the time the Red Cross shelter at the Mississippi Trade Mart had begun to fill with evacuees, many health care volunteers were available to help address medical problems and provide medications, including pharmacists, physicians, and pharmacy students/residents.

From Katrina, we learned of the dire need for services to manage common chronic diseases. The majority of patients seen in our clinics after both hurricanes had many medical problems, no medical insurance, and limited or no ability to purchase medications. We collaborated with the Red Cross and worked closely with the Department of Health to help meet the needs of these evacuees. We now share some personal reflections of our Gustav experience.

Reflections of Amber Holdiness

We opened our disaster relief clinic at the Mississippi Trade Mart, a 25,449-square-foot building, on Labor Day morning. Later that afternoon, Gustav made landfall. Evacuees were bused in, primarily from south Louisiana. My responsibility was to check blood pressures, obtain glucose readings, and take medication histories. One man had a glucose higher than the machine would read. He knew he had diabetes, but he was out of his medications. We gave him insulin and had him return a few hours later. He received insulin injections during the next few days and learned how to self-administer it. I don't know what would have happened had we not been there.

I checked blood pressures using electronic monitors. Several times, I could only get an "error" reading. I was on rotation at the UMMC Hypertension Clinic and had been trained on appropriate blood pressure measurement. One lady who was complaining of headaches said she was out of her medications. I did not realize how hard it would be to get an accurate blood pressure reading under these circumstances. I had the equipment to perform manual blood pressure measurements, but it still took me several attempts to get a reading. Her systolic blood pressure was well over 200 mm Hg. We were able to lower her blood pressure gradually and recheck her during the next few days.

Taking medication histories was the most difficult task I encountered. The population had a low health literacy, and there were often language barriers. There was no way to confirm their medications. I remember talking to one woman with several complaints. She did not know her medications and did not have her bottles. She described one medication as "for my sugar, starts with a G." I determined that she likely was on glyburide. We went through this same lengthy scenario for each of her diseases, and I was finally able to address all of her medication needs. I feel that my patience and vigilance helped get her through the next few days without her complaints developing into an acute circumstance.

Other patients needed more intensive care than we could provide. A lady with cancer needed her chemotherapy. She and her family could not get back to Louisiana and were very distraught. We made many calls and were able to arrange for treatment the next day. I was as relieved as they were. Another man was frantic because he was supposed to receive dialysis that day. We arranged for his dialysis that afternoon. A pregnant girl came in, having contractions 5 minutes apart. We quickly arranged for her to be transported to a nearby hospital. Later, I learned that she and her new baby were doing fine. These patients made me realize how crucial timing and access can be and how the lack of such could have devastating outcomes.

Volunteering at the clinic was a rewarding experience that allowed me to practice clinical skills in a comprehensive manner, counsel and educate patients from very different backgrounds, and work with various types of other health care providers in a challenging environment. The clinic obviously had an impact on those we treated, but I feel I gained so much more. I learned how to communicate better, and I now have much more compassion for those who are displaced. I particularly am now more clearly aware of and grateful for all the opportunities I have had throughout my life.

Reflections of Adam Pate
Hurricane Gustav provided pharmacists and students an exceptional opportunity to care for a vulnerable population. This experience gave me the chance to quickly learn things that textbooks cannot adequately cover. I will never forget my encounter with one lady in particular.

Everything was running smoothly until I sat down with this patient. I quickly recognized that she was ill; she was sweating, fidgeting, and disheveled. Upon questioning, I learned she was in her early 30s, on no medications and with no significant medical history. I thought, "What could be wrong?" Then, I asked if she had ever used illegal drugs. She mumbled and stared at the floor. She seemed embarrassed to respond as I asked again. She then looked up, and I could see the pain in her eyes. She said she used heroin. In that moment, I felt completely useless. What could I do?

I took her for a physician examination. During this time, I looked up heroin withdrawal on my phone and read that clonidine is the mainstay of treatment. I thought, "We will just get her some clonidine and things will be fine." Unfortunately, addiction withdrawal is not that easy.

The patient finished the examination, and we sat down. I explained how medications are supplied and what we would do. She was shivering and told me she was cold. We were backed up with patients, but I felt compelled to stay with her. I searched for a blanket and brought it to her. After ensuring her comfort, I continued with other patients. Periodically, I looked for her. Then, I heard the sound of retching and regurgitation. I saw the blanket on the floor and knew it was her before I rounded the corner and saw her head buried in the garbage can. I tried to comfort her and wrapped the blanket around her vomiting, shivering body. I got her water and stayed with her the rest of the afternoon. The battles of addiction and withdrawal were waging before my eyes.

Eventually, she left, and I did not see her again. I often wonder if she made it home. Is she still fighting addiction? Before, I had little sympathy for those with addiction—their choice, deal with the consequences. I now see the havoc and struggle that ensue. She was in crisis, displaced from whatever home she might have had, and I felt only compassion. I simply gave her a blanket and water, but my mind will never forget.

As a student, I often saw pharmacists view addiction critically. We lose sight of those affected and place a stigma on people getting certain prescriptions. Terminal illness, constant pain, or any number of circumstances may be present. We should not ignore addiction, but as pharmacists, we should think, What can I do to help? Maybe, for starters, simply be open-minded and show that we care enough to know more than just medication profiles.

Reflections of Kristen Pate

As a pharmacy student, I had the opportunity to help evacuees during Hurricane Gustav. As soon as we realized the potential disaster and that people were coming, we immediately began preparation. We spent hours gathering and organizing supplies and medications. We contacted potential volunteers, calling and e-mailing pharmacists and students from every area of practice. A Google Mail account was created to notify volunteers of pivotal planning information. We had a full range of volunteers and were ready to open the doors.

It was surreal to watch the evacuees stepping off the buses. Some were alone; others were with families, from young babies to great-grandparents. We had no idea of their medical needs but knew that many had left home without their medications. It was difficult for me to understand at first why they were not concerned about their medications. Over the next few days, I realized some of their burdens were uncertainties about their families, their homes, and the devastation that was occurring. Bringing their medications was not a priority. All potential victims of a devastating hurricane, they had quickly left everything. This lesson stays with me; patients have real lives, experiencing things beyond what we imagine and concerns other than their medication profile.

My primary roles were recording prescriptions and dispensing medications. I made blank prescriptions and created a recordkeeping system for medications dispensed. My preceptor said it was like practicing pharmacy on a mission trip in an underdeveloped country. Our supplies were limited, so I worked with physicians to select alternatives. I remember one gentleman who was on metoprolol, but we had only nebivolol. I explained the differences and how to take the new β-blocker for his blood pressure. He and most patients were grateful to receive their medications while at the shelter. Patients requesting chronic pain medications were often more difficult to evaluate, and we had limited pain medications. One patient became very frustrated because we did not have the medication he needed. Fortunately, we had made prior arrangements with local pharmacies for patients to get medications not supplied at the clinic.

Students are not typically exposed to such extreme settings, and there is no way to mentally prepare for this kind of experience. Although patient care is emphasized, no pharmacist imagines attempting to comprehensively care for a patient's medical needs while providing the uppermost level of compassion and consolation—because his/her whole life has been turned upside down. There was no way we could truly understand what these people were going through. They handled their emotions differently; some kept to themselves, whereas others seized every opportunity to lament their woes. Many were frantic because of the loss of contact with family members and friends. Hearing these stories over and over allowed me to grow closer to the victims and have empathy for what they were experiencing. They seemed glad just to have someone listen. This was a wonderful experience for me. I was able to grow closer to my fellow students and preceptor on an entirely different level, and I truly feel that I was able to make a difference in the lives of many people during a troubled time. It was refreshing to see how many pharmacists and students were also eager to volunteer.

Reflections of Deborah Minor

Our post-hurricane experiences reflect why I decided to enter the profession of pharmacy. I entered pharmacy because of a community pharmacist and his insight. He made me realize that being a pharmacist would always open doors for me in community service. Hundreds of patients benefited from the care provided in our disaster relief clinics, and my pharmacy students had the chance to experience a different side of health care and pharmacy education. They saw the attitudes of service and dedication that flow so freely in our profession, the immediate response to those in need, the thoughtful planning that goes into ensuring that each patient need is met in a stressful environment, and the feeling of "community" working closely with pharmacists from other various areas of practice and other health care providers. It refreshed the spirit of professionalism and service that motivates most health care providers to choose careers in the healing professions. These pharmacy students brought credit to themselves and to the profession.

Reflections During Hurricane Katrina

Ann McMahon Wicker, Pharm.D., BCPS
Clinician

The world is changing very quickly; however, many things remain the same. People will become ill, and skilled health care providers will continue to be in demand.

Scientific and technological advances are occurring at an astounding pace. Computers, BlackBerries, iPhones, iPads, etc., assist pharmacists in providing critical care to patients. We have come to greatly use these instruments in rendering care. However, we must remember the motto of the Boy Scouts of America—Be prepared.

We all have dreams—some pleasant, others horrific, and many, professionally related nightmares.

I dream that winds are blowing and waters are rising at the hospital. To complicate matters, the clinical pharmacy manager has a wound on her leg. However, there is no time for self-pity, for three buses of patients being evacuated from the hospital are in need of 4 days of prescriptions (oral and IV). The pharmacists use teamwork to fill the prescriptions. Additionally, they move the pharmacy to the second floor to escape the rising waters and continue their commitment to care for the 62 remaining patients. A closet on the second floor becomes the pharmacy, piled high, stuffed with bins of drugs on cafeteria trays for shelving. Fortunately, institutions such as the University of Louisiana at Monroe, Xavier University, and Ochsner Health System instill commitment to care for others, self-determination, mental toughness, attention to detail, and teamwork in their professionals. Thank goodness that mentors taught innovation.

Power is lost, rendering all power-driven devices useless. Be prepared. The situation becomes chaotic, but there is no time for complaining. The waters on the first floor must be navigated to obtain any additional medicine to sustain patients. Teamwork is necessary, especially since the wounded pharmacist must exercise caution to avoid the infectious waters. A gurney becomes a navigational vessel. Agility, skills, and the dedication of the team result in obtaining their goal (medications).

The nightmare continues. Approximately 200 refugees are brought by boat to the hospital. The team continues filling prescriptions and counseling patients. Team members rotate naps at night on the roof of the hospital to escape the heat. The situation is overwhelming; however, the team is relentless in its commitment. Drug therapies must be changed to preserve a depleting inventory.

Information is scarce from a flooded city. The team is informed that patients will be moved to a makeshift MASH unit on the third floor of the city jail. Thugs are on the prowl in the neighborhood, and they are seeking drugs from any source.

The word circulates to be prepared for rescue, even though no one knows when that will happen. A sponge bath with the leftover rainwater on the roof provides temporary relief.

Finally, the sound of Chinook helicopters is music to the team's ears. The sight of a hospital immersed in 15 feet of water wakes me from my dream.

I thank God that it is only a nightmare of my recollection on my 5-day, 4-night war story as a clinical pharmacy manager at Chalmette Medical Center in Chalmette, Louisiana, during Hurricane Katrina in August 2005.

End-of-Life Care

Rebecca A. Taylor, Pharm.D., MBA, BCPS
Clinician

I was working as the clinical pharmacist on a Wednesday in September when we received a consult for Mrs. Q's hydromorphone PCA and "itching issues." This was not a typical pharmacist consult, but every now and then in our small community hospital, we were asked to review complex cases for pain or TPN or cases for underinsured patients. I reviewed the medical record and began to learn the story of Mrs. Q, a woman in her 50s who was suffering from metastatic neuroendocrine cancer and experiencing severe flushing reactions as a result. She had scratched open her skin on many occasions and had tried a myriad of antihistamines, creams, and corticosteroids. Unfortunately, I happened to know quite a bit about neuroendocrine cancer, as my 42-year-old uncle was suffering from the same disease process. I had spent countless weeknights and weekends researching octreotide depot, oxaliplatin reactions (he had profound neuropathy), and remedies for flushing associated with neuroendocrine cancer.

I went in to see Mrs. Q and her family right away. Her husband was a railroad engineer, and she had two teenagers in high school. She led a simple life and worked at the local library. I took a careful history of her pain medication use (she was up to oxycodone 600 mg every 24 hours with multiple breakthrough regimes). The physicians had attempted to convert her to hydromorphone PCA on admission. As I sat and listened to the patient's history, I couldn't keep the images of my uncle out of my head. My uncle was a thin man to start with, but then he just kept losing weight. We tried everything: steroids, Marinol, Ensure, Remeron, protein shakes. Nothing worked. The nausea was tremendous, and he just kept losing weight. Mrs. Q weighed about 90 pounds. What a terrible disease to be afflicted with, and how awful to have so little understanding of how, why, and what treatments could actually mitigate it. My aunt spent and still spends 3–4 hours a day searching the Internet for clinical trials, joining support groups, researching radioisotopes for neuroendocrine cancer. It envelops every conversation I have with her. She is one of my closest family members. The cancer has changed our family. Every call is a possibility of more bad news, more metastases, more failed treatments, side effects from tyrosine kinase inhibitors, ruling out a new infection. It's just exhausting. I could relate to this family. I could see what they'd been through, and I knew it all too well. When a smoker is struck with lung cancer, although it is unfortunate, at least there is a reasonable cause. Neuroendocrine cancer is very poorly understood by health care professionals, let alone patients. They asked about the itching. I attempted to explain the reasons for the flushing, saying that it was thought to be related to hormone release and an increase in histamine and serotonin in the tissues. Mrs. Q was currently on diphenhydramine 50 mg orally every 6 hours with little to no relief.

I walked into the room, and Mrs. Q asked me to sit down next to her bed. I asked her to describe the flushing and asked about what she'd tried in the past. She described rushes of heat, discomfort, and annoying, constant itching. She said it felt like "there was a fire raging through the top layer of her skin." I took a complete medication history, including allergies. I thanked her for her time and promised to be back with a plan in a short while. I left the room a little choked up. I recalled that, on my first clinical rotation as an APPE student, we used cyproheptadine in the BMT patients who were experiencing itching. I thought it was worth a try. I also tailored the hydromorphone PCA with an appropriate basal rate and demand dosage. After the orders were written, I went in to speak with the family. They were extremely grateful for the new option of a medication for the itching. I could tell this was a very big quality-of-life issue. I checked in with her the next morning, and her itching symptoms had decreased by about 50 percent! I couldn't believe it. I was so proud and so happy to assist in a small portion of her care. To most, itching may be considered a relatively minor side effect, but in a patient with a ticking time clock, it can be the difference between making her teenager's soccer game or not. I wanted to be part of the solution for Mrs. Q and her family.

They received news later that week that her chemotherapeutic options were waning, and I saw an order come through the pharmacy order system for comfort care measures only. I went to visit the family shortly after, and Mrs. Q held my hand for about 5 minutes. She looked relieved as the itching had subsided and as the hydromorphone PCA was turned up to 2 mg/hour. I thanked everyone for letting us provide her care and gave my business card to her husband. He hugged me on the way out. I had a feeling I might never see this patient again.

I saw the obituary later in the month, but the family requested a small service of immediate family members only. A few weeks later, a thank you card appeared in my mailbox. I assumed it was from a recent IPPE student we had on rotations with us, and I opened it, as I would have any other official work mail. I was wrong. The letter was from Mr. Q, thanking me for allowing his wife to pass in peace and for all of the assistance we provided for her in the last few days of her life. I couldn't believe it! It was my first letter from a patient, and I started to cry. I thought about Mrs. Q and about how handling her issues took up just a small part of my day, but apparently, it was a large part of her day. A small excerpt from the letter read, "Thank you for helping us in our time of need. Your knowledge and caring helped my wife make it through her last days. We are forever grateful...."

This one small intervention did not change the patient's outcome or save the hospital thousands of dollars, but the knowledge that I improved her quality of life helped me better understand our professional duty to tend to patients' needs. Pharmacy can feel thankless, especially on those days of desperation and back-to-back meetings. Memories of people like Mrs. Q remind me that our greatest duty is to take care of patients, one at a time. Perhaps it is an impromptu counseling session at the out-window that improves a patient's ability to adhere to her inhaler, a discussion about moving the timing of medications to make it more convenient, or changing an antihistamine so a patient can die in peace without itching. These lessons are best shared with those we mentor: residents, students, interns. I try to impart the importance of listening, having patience, and being creative in problem solving with those I teach. I'm grateful to have met Mrs. Q and her family.

Care Across Cultures

Multicultural Awareness

If we are to achieve a richer culture, rich in contrasting values, we must recognize the whole gamut of human potentialities, and so weave a less arbitrary social fabric, one in which each diverse human gift will find a fitting place.

Margaret Mead

A physician is obligated to consider more than a diseased organ, more even than the whole man—he must view the man in his world.

Harvey Cushing

The Cultural Dimensions of Patient Care in Alaska

Jane McLaughlin-Middlekauff, Pharm.D.
Educator

A young Alaska Native child sits down with a parent in the pediatric pharmacy and looks at me as I interview her mother, verifying the child's name, date of birth, weight, allergies, and over-the-counter usage. I look up and notice the child's continued examination of me; the child whispers to her mother, and I proceed to ask if everything is okay. The mother smiles and states that her daughter has never before seen anyone with curly hair and green eyes in the remote Alaskan village where they live.

Growing up in the small town of Thornton, Iowa, with a population of 424 people, I did not have a vast amount of diversity. After experiencing the inquisitive eyes of the Alaska Native child, I began to question how I looked at those who were different from me. Did I gaze too long at others? Was I unintentionally making assumptions about the person based on the person's address, age, appearance, or enrolled/documented tribal enrollment? It was not until my husband, Aaron, received military orders to be stationed at Elmendorf Air Force Base in Anchorage, Alaska, that I would experience and learn about how a life lived elsewhere could vary so much.

During my first week at Alaska Native Medical Center (ANMC) at Southcentral Foundation (SCF), I attended orientation, which included something I had never before encountered, cultural training. This was an amazing eye-opening experience to Alaska Natives (who are employed by SCF) discussing their own personal or family experiences based on topics such as health care, education, tribal traditions, cultural aspects all staff should be aware of, and how best to care for the patient population. Never before had I been cautioned not to discuss a medication for the patient's particular disease state. Instead, pharmacists and other health care providers were to refer to a medication in general terms, such as "This medication is for *our* diabetes" or "This medication is for diabetes," and avoid stating, "This medication is for *your* diabetes." Pharmacists were cautioned to avoid personalizing or implying ownership of a disease state to an Alaska Native patient when providing pharmaceutical counseling.

Hearing stories about culture from Alaska Natives was a very moving experience at orientation, but it wasn't until I was fully engaged in the social and working environment that I learned about the health care risks, on which our teams of health care providers (including a pharmacist) would be responsible for educating patients. Indeed, educating Alaska Native patients on medications and diet provided a new perspective as they taught me about their native way of life, Alaska Native history, and pride in their traditional cultures. For instance, the lack of literature regarding medication interactions with Alaska native food (e.g., seal oil, muktuk) made recommendations and counseling more challenging when investigating the cause of an INR out of range or a possible food-drug interaction. I was challenged to think critically and handle public health issues as they arose. For example, I quickly learned that it couldn't be assumed that everyone was aware of the tooth decay associated with placing soda pop in a propped-up baby bottle. Similarly, ikmik (a combination of either dried tobacco leaves or regular tobacco chew mixed with a form of fungus found on some Alaskan trees) should not be used to soothe teething babies.

In addition, providing pharmaceutical care services to patients across the different remote villages presented challenges for communication and cooperation. Along with caring for pediatric patients, I had many opportunities to teach, engage with, and learn from all ages of Alaska Native patients in the anticoagulation clinic and ambulatory pharmacy. Previously, I had monitored patients in anticoagulation clinics in the lower 48 states, but it wasn't until I took care of anticoagulation patients across the vast land mass of Alaska that I truly comprehended the obstacles with blood draws and food supplies. In the lower 48 states, I had been accustomed to receiving lab results in a very timely manner without much coordination of effort. When we needed a blood sample from a patient living on an Alaskan island or remote area (which required a bush plane to transport the blood sample), new obstacles were introduced involving fog and snow, which would keep the bush plane from landing or taking off from the airstrip. Coordinating the efforts of the anticoagulation clinic, the health aide in the village to draw the blood sample, the bush pilot, and the patient required dedication and communication by everyone involved. Realizing the challenges faced by Alaska Native patients on a regular basis and the diversity of the population that I had been given the opportunity to serve as an ambulatory pediatric pharmacist at ANMC brought defining moments in my career.

These experiences strengthened my learning and decision-making skills to consider limitations that could affect future decisions when developing plans or goals. Patients living in remote villages or on an Alaskan island faced obstacles regarding the availability of food and supplies. For instance, for patients from remote villages, there were few options for transportation. Before suggesting changes to a patient's diet, I had to fully understand the food situation of the area. What was the situation for patients living on an Alaskan island who might depend on fishing, hunting, and gathering berries and eggs for the majority of their meals? Or what was the situation for others who might need to purchase their food and household supplies a year in advance and receive them from an annual barge to avoid severely overpriced groceries at their local small store? As you can imagine, obtaining supplies and food in villages that are reachable only by dog sled, snow machine, four-wheeler, boat, or bush plane can be quite difficult.

Educating patients as well as pharmacy students on rotation with me has been a passion of mine since I graduated from Drake University. As the pharmacy student rotation coordinator at SCF, I believed that the cultural aspect of practicing pharmacy should begin with opportunities to develop an understanding of Alaska Native culture not only by attending cultural training, but also by learning about tribal medicine by traditional healers. After building a working relationship with one of the tribal medicine healers and the director of traditional medicine (Dr. Ted Mala), I arranged for each pharmacy student on rotation at ANMC to meet with him to gain clarity about and coherence of the relationship between tribal and Western medicine. The opportunity to learn more about integrative medicine, tribal medicine, talking circles, and the way of life in remote villages assisted in the cultural development of pharmacist students who had never been exposed to this culture. Also important in their development was the application of what they had learned by communicating with patients. Students were cautioned about their use of nonverbal communication when speaking with Alaska Native patients. Patients could recognize the movement of eyebrows, body placement/movement, eye contact, and tone of voice to tell the story of what a person was thinking or feeling. The pharmacy students were excited to reflect on their understanding of the Alaska Native culture and the ways in which tribal doctors are incorporated in a patient's plan. Some students wrote final reflections of their experiences that were published in their university newsletter or presented at their respective college of pharmacy. Rotation students encouraged others to seek out these unique experiences to better prepare themselves for their future in the profession of pharmacy, which serves diverse populations.

After 6 years in Alaska, my husband and I received notice we were to be stationed in Miami, Florida. The experiences I gained while serving Alaska Native patients involved my development into a more culturally sensitive person, which has served me well in the population of South Florida, which is very diverse culturally. Working with students on rotation at ANMC helped me create pedagogical methods to educate future pharmacists about the importance of communication (verbal and nonverbal) in the development of patient understanding. My interest in working with a diverse population has evolved into my participation in clinical research, looking at health disparities in relation to a culturally diverse population. I will always remember the wonderful opportunity I gleaned from patients while working on teams with outstanding health care providers and staff. These patients clarified and molded my understanding of how best to serve and embrace the patient population of Alaska Natives. In a world full of different races and cultures, it is imperative that pharmacists be open-minded to diversity and trained on how to be a culturally sensitive professional.

Diamonds in the Dust

Betty Ann Torres, Pharm.D.
Educator/Clinician

Frances M. Rodríguez, Pharm.D., BCPS
Educator/Clinician

It was an active morning in the Ambulatory Gynecology Clinic at our academic, tertiary medical center of the University of Puerto Rico; this was the day we cared for girls and adolescents. The cloudy weather made me think about how, on this particular day, we tried to help these young patients and their parents/custodians navigate through gray clouds of information related to diseases, medications, pregnancy, or sexual abuse.

As part of the interdisciplinary team, I, the clinical pharmacist, make pharmaceutical care interventions for the girls and the parents/custodians before the patient sees the gynecologist. This day, however, the task at hand was not as sad or worrisome as a sexual abuse case or a too-early-in-life pregnancy. As I entered the evaluation room, I saw a mother and her 3-year-old little girl waiting for the initial interview. The mother's eyes glanced at me apprehensively when she gave me, a pharmacist, a referral from the pediatrician: assessment and treatment of labial adhesion. The mother probably thought, "What could be so wrong that even the pharmacist needs to see my girl."

The mother's demeanor showed extreme concern and nervousness. She told me in a low voice that something bad was happening to her daughter. As a Hispanic mother, I could understand her despair in thinking that her girl could have a condition or defect in her reproductive system, which is something that, culturally, we should not discuss because, as a girl, her body should be pristine and intact. As a Hispanic professional, I know that little information on reproductive issues is discussed with patients. There is a tendency to avoid this uncomfortable topic.

As I proceeded with the usual interview process, I began to ask rather mechanically about the patient's general health as well as the presence of common pediatric diseases and any other conditions. When I asked about pediatric immunizations, the mother looked at me in a defensive manner and said: "My child's vaccinations are current. I am a very cautious mother! I do not know how this happened! What can I do to protect my little girl?"

Lots of questions immediately filled my mind. How many girls are referring to this clinic with the same condition? How are these Hispanic mothers handling the news? Are they receiving the information in the way a Hispanic mother will understand? As if reflexively, I found myself saying: "Ma'am, I am going to be with you and your girl in this process. As soon as the gynecologist sees you, we will meet again in my office, and we will start all over again but in a different tone."

This type of referral should not be done in a routine, matter-of-fact way. I felt the responsibility and commitment to help take care of the situation by breaking the common patterns of pharmacy interventions in this clinic. As a clinical pharmacist, I know that my responsibility is to assess any drug-related problems before the gynecologist sees the patients so that these problems are accounted for when the patient's pharmacotherapy is discussed and the prescriptions are written. As a result, I see the patient only once. However, our clinics are so busy and the fiscal resources are so limited that the interdisciplinary team always welcomes a helping hand, even if it crosses a little bit the different disciplines' boundaries. Usually, the physician will explain the condition and the social worker will deal with the emotional aspect if not too occupied with the worst cases.

When we had the chance to meet again, I spoke to her as a mother who happens to be a health professional. The tone of our conversation was different, informative but different. I emphasized that her little girl was not different from other girls because of this condition—that she, as a mother, had done nothing wrong. She was not careless; on the contrary, she looked for help—even when taking such a young girl to the gynecologist could be frowned on. I carefully inserted bits of education among my reassurance and empathic words.

She could see that I was able to take time to understand her at different levels, emotionally and culturally. She could also see that, as a pharmacist, I was there not only to explain and educate on the particulars of the medication therapy from behind the barrier of a counter, but also, as a concerned health professional, to help patients as a whole. At the end of our interview, her *"me siento mejor, vamos a estar bien"* ("I feel better, we will be okay") was good confirmation for me.

Later, the gynecologist came to me and acknowledged the contribution I had made to change this patient's experience for the better. She also said: "I urge you to keep working with this patient population as referrals are increasing."

As pharmacists, we can go further in our profession: impressing other professionals and patients with our versatility and having an impact on specific populations and their diverse way of thinking. All we need is to seek opportunities and have a commitment to change gray clouds for white ones. We need to be diamonds in the dust that can be the health care system. Pharmacists have the knowledge, the disposition, and the accessibility to be active components of the multidisciplinary health care team.

Back to Basics:
Reflection on a Medical Mission

Kristin Held, Pharm.D., BCOP
Clinician

When a physician first invited me on a medical mission to Palestine, I thought he was joking. He wasn't. He had been contacted by a nonprofit organization to select a medical team to survey the current pediatric oncology services in the outlying areas of Palestine. Our team consisted of a physician, nurse, nurse practitioner, social worker, and myself—a clinical pharmacy specialist in pediatric stem cell transplant. Although I had completed a PGY2 specialty residency 1 year earlier, I wondered if I was qualified for such a task. The experience in a region with limited resources, variations in training levels, and different cultural perspectives caused me to focus back on the basics, which I had lost sight of in my preoccupation with drug therapy. As pharmacists, we become engrossed in the pharmacologic treatment of various conditions and sometimes overlook the basic principles or management strategies. This was my opportunity to integrate the experiences that I had gained working at various oncology programs into helping to build a new facility and into educating the staff to ensure a safe environment for pediatric oncology patients.

When I was preparing for the trip, I outlined important aspects of oncology pharmacy practice including pertinent reference materials and educational topics. As I reviewed my notes, I quickly realized that what I was missing were the general principles. After further evaluation of my training, where I started learning the basics of oncology practice, I chose to focus on the safe handling of chemotherapy and the identification and management of oncologic emergencies.

We were invited to visit three hospitals during our week abroad and asked to assess the current clinical pediatric oncology services of each. The majority of our time was spent at a government hospital that was accessible to approximately 90 percent of the pediatric oncology population. As we walked through the hospital, our team was shocked by the neglected condition of the facility and by their lack of resources. I asked to see the designated area for chemotherapy preparation and was pleasantly surprised to see a functioning hood located in a separate room on the adult oncology unit. After taking a closer look, however, I quickly realized that the hood surfaces were visibly contaminated. The condition of the chemotherapy preparation area strengthened my original goal to pare down the information I provided to the general principles that could be built upon through further education and experience.

Following the tour, we were given time to sit with the staff in order to identify topics of interest for discussion. Extravasation was quickly identified by both physicians and nurses as a significant complication in this patient population. Once the group was collected, I was amazed by the size of the audience. The seating was limited in the back office and staff members huddled together on a couch on one side of the room. Many chairs were brought into the room to form a semicircle around the computer desk where I sat. I was inundated with questions shortly after I began to discuss the topic on my prepared slides. As a pharmacist, I anticipated questions regarding drug therapy, and I quickly realized that the medications we use in the United States to manage extravasations were unavailable. As I was preparing the presentation, I had not considered this! The nurse practitioner and I salvaged the discussion by focusing on the identification and initial management of a potential extravasation. We encouraged the group to openly discuss current monitoring strategies for patients receiving potential vesicants and evaluated how this could be improved. The conversation quickly changed directions and the nursing staff discussed their lack of confidence in ensuring bloodflow with central venous catheters. The open forum provided us an opportunity to reassure the nurses by scheduling time to observe and provide hands-on training related to accessing and flushing port-a-caths before our departure.

At the end of the presentation, I was self-conscious that the presentation had not gone as intended. Despite these feelings of inadequacy, I received praise from the physician who had invited me on the mission trip as well as from many attendees, who hoped to directly relate the information they received to patients. This was only one instance in which I felt that I positively affected the care of patients in this underserved area. Although the topics that I focused on during the trip did not require critical evaluation of the primary literature related to a novel drug therapy as it often does in preparation for a lecture in my everyday practice, the fundamentals that I reviewed during the trip were vital to safe and effective management of pediatric oncology patients. I am confident that these principles will become the framework for a successful program as the nurses and physicians continue to practice within the setting. The greatest asset that I identified during this journey was the experiences I was provided through both experiential rotations and residency training. By taking myself back to where I began as a technician with an interest in oncology and through my experiences as a trained clinical specialist, I was able to identify and teach the necessary elements to foster the future development of clinical skills.

Learning Beyond a Classroom Setting: Study Abroad Experience in Traditional Chinese Medicine

Courtney L. Tam, Pharm.D.
Student

S tepping onto a public bus in Guangzhou, China, I was heading toward Sun Yat-Sen University Cancer Center (SUCC) to complete a rotation focusing on Traditional Chinese Medicine (TCM). Having arrived the previous day from New York City, I was still in disbelief and wonderment that I had chosen to travel to the other side of the world to complete a rotation at such a prestigious hospital. Walking into SUCC, I found that those feelings slowly intermingled with nervousness. Over the course of the next few weeks, I experienced many new things and developed an understanding of "pharmacy" through another country's culture.

Existing for more than 5,000 years, TCM is commonly used within the Chinese population.[1] It is an ancient holistic medical system whose goals are "to identify and treat the root cause of conditions so that the healing is genuine and the condition does not recur."[2] Traditional Chinese medicine is considered complementary and alternative medicine (CAM) in the United States. It encompasses a variety of therapies including Chinese herbal medicine, acupuncture, cupping, and *tui na* (Chinese massage).[2, 3]

A typical day in the TCM pharmacy at SUCC includes a lecture from one of the herbal pharmacists on the different classes of herbs and their uses and on the filling of herbal prescriptions. The pharmacists would teach me how to use a brass scale and how to counsel patients on different ways to prepare the herbal decoction. I was astonished at how many prescriptions the TCM pharmacy was able to fill—about 2,000 a day. Most of the TCM prescriptions were handwritten, and if handwritten prescriptions in New York City are sometimes hard to read, Chinese handwritten prescriptions by comparison are several times more illegible. This increased my appreciation of electronic prescriptions.

The prescriptions are usually written for a mix of different herbal products to be used as a decoction. The procedure reminded me of when I would go with my friends to buy candy at Dylan's Candy Bar. Like the candy aisle at this store, the cabinet containing the herbs aligned them in a row. I would take a scoop of herbs with my hand and measure it on a scale. Usually, I would repeat this with five or more different herbs depending on the prescription. I even got to grab handfuls of dried scorpions, snakes, water bugs, and centipedes. The most shocking Chinese herb, one that I never thought would be considered for medicinal use, is *si gua luo*, luffa vegetable sponge. *Si gua luo* uses include eliminating toxins and dissolving phlegm, stopping bleeding, and alleviating stiffness.[1] The pharmacists made jokes stating that the Chinese used it to wash dishes. I remember exactly what I was thinking, "I use it to exfoliate my skin. Now I can make it into some sort of decoction to drink? Ewww." I would mix the herbs (much like a child mixing his gummy worms and other candies) in a pan and then evenly separate the mixture into different envelopes. The final mixture is checked by a pharmacist. This whole process is fascinating to witness, yet it allowed me to realize how difficult, cumbersome, and confusing a treatment regimen can be for a patient, especially if the patient has more than one prescription.

Another interesting discovery in the TCM pharmacy was the supply of herbal medications that were already compounded in dosage forms resembling Western medications (e.g., such as tablets, capsules, patches). Some were considered over-the-counter (OTC) formulations and were labeled as such, much like the prepackaged OTC medications in New York. This was intriguing to me because I was not aware that herbal medications came in these dosage formulations. I assume these dosage forms helped with patient adherence, since there would be no need for the patient to clean the raw herbs and perform the 1-hour boiling procedure to prepare a decoction at home.

The community pharmacies in Guangzhou were in some ways similar to pharmacies in New York City, but in others, they were extremely different. Most of the retail pharmacies would sell Western medications (e.g., Claritin® and Tylenol®). They would also sell Chinese herbal medications, for prescription or OTC use. There, I got to see herbal medications that the hospital might not carry, such as dried geckos, dried human placenta, and dried seahorses. Each of these has its own unique medicinal use; for example, the dried human placenta can be used to nourish blood, especially in postpartum women.[1] What I found scandalous was how some of the Chinese pharmacies worked; they would sell prescription medications, Western medications (e.g., antibiotics, blood pressure medications, and smoking cessation drugs) and certain Chinese herbals (e.g., antibiotics), without a prescription. According to the pharmacists at SUCC, this is a common practice, especially with antibiotics, even though prescriptions are necessary for these medications, because going to see a doctor is expensive in China, and most of the time, patients have to pay out of their own pockets. As a future pharmacist and health care professional, I worry about the common antibiotic abuse and resistance.[4] Even more appalling, counseling is rarely offered in Guangzhou community pharmacies, even though the pharmacy may not be busy.

Aside from visiting pharmacies, I got the chance to learn about TCM therapies firsthand. As mentioned earlier, TCM is a holistic system; thus, some people use such therapies to maintain homeostasis of their body and possibly prevent future ailments. My most memorable experience is with cupping, which is used for diseases such as gastrointestinal issues or headaches.[5] Cupping consists of applying a heated cup to the skin and certain acupuncture points. The reduced pressure in the cup draws in the skin, holding the cup in place. The cup may be moved while the suction is taking place, causing a "regional pulling" of the muscle and skin. Cupping helps open up the skin's pores and "stimulate[s] the flow of blood, balances and realigns the flow of qi, breaks up obstructions, and creates an avenue for toxins to be drawn out of the body."[6] I went to a TCM medical clinic for cupping with a friend who had had it done before and said that it felt good; she mentioned that some people get addicted to it. She went first and looked comfortable during the funny, yet interesting-looking procedure. I can only summarize my experience with the proverb, "Curiosity killed the cat." I let my back be the guinea pig. The heated cup was placed on it, and a variant cupping technique involving sliding was performed; I cried out in pain. Trying to recapture my suave composure, I decided to opt for the regular cupping. Bad decision: my back ended up with black bruises, some of which were painless. I was told that the bruises were normal and that the reason mine were so dark was because my body has "wetness" (not literal or physical wetness); the cupping, I was told, was removing the cold and "wetness" from my body. Apparently, I can get this "wetness" and cold from the food I eat. The spots disappeared eventually, but it took awhile. Would I recommend cupping? Based on this experience, not really, plus the literature out there does not support its use in curing any disease.[7]

The TCM rotation allowed me to acquire knowledge and hands-on experience in an area of pharmacy, herbal medicine, which I would never be able to gain in a classroom setting. It made me more appreciative of the convenience of Western medications, such as the ease of swallowing a tablet, the rules and regulations the United States has on the standardization of prescription products and OTC medications, and the routine practice of counseling patients on their medications. Although I see advantages to Western pharmacy and its practices, I value the holistic emphasis TCM strives to achieve, which is to treat the underlying problem, unlike Western medicine, which often is focused on treating the symptoms of the disease. Overall, the cultural exchange and learning opportunities that occurred throughout the rotation were definitely valuable, and I would strongly recommend that future students study abroad if they get the opportunity.

I wish to express my sincere gratitude to Dr. Zhe-Sheng Chen and Dr. Li-Wu Fu for making this TCM rotation at Sun Yat-Sen University Cancer Center possible. I'd also like to thank Marie George for encouraging me to share this experience with others.

1. National Center for Complementary and Alternative Medicine. Available at www.nccam.nih.gov/. Accessed September 13, 2011.
2. Traditional Chinese Medicine World Foundation. Available at www.tcmworld.org/. Accessed September 13, 2011.
3. Traditional Chinese Medicine Resource Center. Available at www.tcmcentral.com/. Accessed September 13, 2011.
4. Yung J. The Chinese Government's Antibiotics Crackdown. Global Post. 2009. Available at www.globalpost.com/dispatch/china/091209/stockpiling-antibiotics?page=0,0. Accessed September 13, 2011.

5. Dharmananda S. Cupping. Institute for Traditional Medicine. Available at www.itmonline. org/arts/cupping.htm#figure. Accessed September 13, 2011.

6. Cupping. Acupuncture Today. Available at www.acupuncturetoday.org/abc/cupping.php. Accessed September 13, 2011.

7. Cupping. American Cancer Society. 2008. Available at www.cancer.org/Treatment/TreatmentsandSideEffects/ComplementaryandAlternativeMedicine/HerbsVitaminsandMinerals/cupping?sitearea=ETO. Accessed September 13, 2011.

The Homeless and Health Care

Robert Draeger, Pharm.D.
Clinician

W hen my daughter was young, we went to a festival not very
far from home on a beautiful fall day. Unfortunately, upon
arrival, my daughter managed to close her fingers in the car door. I
quickly got the door open, and as she looked at me through teary
eyes, she said, "I just want to go home." I often think of this incident
when I see the homeless patients in our clinics and remember the
phrases "Home sweet home," "Home is where the heart is," and
"There is no place like home." Sadly, today, more people are finding
themselves on the verge of homelessness; a lost job, a few missed
mortgage payments, and suddenly you are on the street. Hopefully,
you have friends or relatives to help. Others may not be so lucky,
and they end up in a shelter—or worse, living in their car or on the
street. The comforts of home are gone.

The media often portray the homeless as dirty, odoriferous,
clothed in rags, and carrying their worldly possessions in a large trash
bag—suffering from alcoholism, drug abuse, or mental illness. Often,
it may be assumed they live on the street, in an abandoned building,
under a bridge, or in a bug-infested shelter. None of this should de-
prive them of basic health care. But where do such people go for this
care? Access to care may be available in a free or public clinic, the
emergency room of a local hospital—or nowhere at all. Even though
there may be access to care, getting to the site of care can be a major
issue. Treatment is most likely rapid, but follow-up may be difficult or
impossible. The homeless patient returns to the streets, while other
patients return to the comfort of their homes.

What about the choice of treatment or "guidelines" for treating
the homeless? Here are a few examples of issues I have encountered
in my follow-ups of homeless patients. A patient with hypertension
is started on a diuretic. He or she has no bathroom but does find a
secluded alley and ends up being arrested for urinating in public. An
infection is treated with an antibiotic that is to be taken three times

a day with food—a regimen that is difficult to follow when you don't know the next time you will have food to eat. In addition, there is the possible side effect of diarrhea. A patient treated with a drug that has sedative side effects sleeps soundly and wakes up to find that all of his or her belongings have been stolen. Then there is the person with diabetes who is given insulin and syringes. Where is a refrigerator? How safe is it to walk the streets with a bag of syringes? Or maybe this diabetic patient is fortunate enough to live in a shelter where they serve donuts and juice in the morning and pasta, bread, corn, rice, and potatoes for the other meals: a diet that will do wonders for blood sugar control. When one selects a drug regimen, it is based on known outcomes, with normal adherence issues. Homeless patients may not fit the norm because of their special living situations.

I consider myself fortunate to be able to interact with the homeless population in my current position with the college of pharmacy. I am able to practice at five inner-city clinics, taking students on rotations with me and focusing on a patient population with a very special problem: "homelessness." In addition, these patients may have many health issues, no insurance, and little or no money. It is not the typical population our students see, nor is it one they often think about. Through their exposure to it, students are able to understand the unique treatment issues of the homeless and learn to practice their profession by serving all members of society. Often, these students volunteer at the drop-in center after their rotation, realizing the needs of the patients and the self-fulfillment gained from being involved with them. I believe that, through their exposure to the homeless, students will continue to work toward solving the problems of health care in the homeless.

The Amazing Mr. M: "It took me 88 years, but I finally got to college"

Erica Estus, Pharm.D., CGP
Educator

Three years ago, I was introduced to Mr. M during my first semester as a faculty member at the University of Rhode Island (URI) College of Pharmacy, teaching a geriatric pharmacotherapy elective. My idea was to take the twenty-two P2 students enrolled in the course out of the classroom so that they could interact with older adults through various site visit activities. I asked the activities director from a local senior residential community to recruit three older adult volunteers to work with three students who were planning to come to administer fall risk assessments. And then, in walked Mr. M...and life has never been the same.

On the first day of class that first semester, when I asked my students about their previous interactions with older adults, many said they had only interacted with their grandparents. And those who had spent time with older adults described negative experiences from the community pharmacy setting. It quickly became apparent that these students needed some positive interactions with the elderly to alter some of the negative perceptions—and that this was not going to happen in the classroom using traditional methods.

Upon being introduced to Mr. M, I found him warm and funny. He began to joke with the two other men who had volunteered to help the three pharmacy students administer the fall risk tool. Initially, however, the encounter was awkward, and I began to think that my idea of taking students off-campus to learn was not very good. But then, Mr. M worked his magic...he answered every question on the fall risk assessment accurately and without hesitation. And when it was time to demonstrate his gait, he literally jumped up, eager to do so. Mr. M proceeded to poke fun at the other two volunteers because he "outscored" them, and to his delight, this was a sore spot for one of them. At the time, Mr. M was 88, and the students could not believe how amazingly spry he was for his age. They stated in their written reflections that they had never met anyone like him. His energy, enthusiasm, and "zest" for life made the students want to return to the facility—and they did, with their friends.

The activities at the senior residential community continued and expanded—pharmacy students working with older adults, playing the Wii, teaching computer skills, holding wellness fairs, and even planning a "senior" prom—all strategies to improve communication between students and older adults. Providing opportunities to build relationships between students and elderly people removed communication barriers between two generations that often don't understand each other. Residents of this senior living community grew accustomed to having the URI pharmacy students there regularly during service learning experiences, advanced pharmacy practice experiences, outreach opportunities through the student ASCP (American Society of Consultant Pharmacists) chapter, and the geriatric elective.

Mr. M continued to interact with the pharmacy students whenever possible. He really captured their interest by his passion for investing. A self-taught investor, he started his own "investment club" at the senior living community. He never attended college, but he easily knew more about stocks and dividends than many people on Wall Street. Pharmacy students were always amazed by what they learned in 1 hour with him, and they took more notes at one of his investment club sessions than during an entire pharmacology lecture.

Last year, several residents from this senior living community sent the graduating pharmacy students a video message, which I delivered at the URI graduation banquet. Mr. M had some words of advice he couldn't wait to share: "First paycheck you get, start taking something right off the top, and put it away forever. And if you do that all of your life, you'll be okay." And since that is probably not taught in a pharmacoeconomics course, it was a perfect lesson for Mr. M to share with these pharmacy students.

Mr. M has visited the URI campus a few times to participate in the geriatric elective, and I still remember the spring in his step when I dropped him off after class his first day. "It took me 88 years, but I finally got to college," he said. One November, he presented a special Veterans Day session, telling the pharmacy students about life overseas during World War II and showing them detailed maps of the area he covered while serving in the military. Students also learned about the special relationship he had with his wife—how he cared for her while she suffered from Alzheimer disease—and they discussed the challenges of affording nursing home care.

But the real issue with the students was that Mr. M took only two medications. They just couldn't understand how that was possible "at his age." So they would spend the allotted time just talking with him, almost forgetting about the interview task, but instead learning how he manages his gout—and how he takes apple cider vinegar along with honey every day (and swears by it, as he has done for most of his life). He volunteered to be a patient for the P3 patient assessment workshop so that students could practice taking blood pressure and interview him about any medication-related problems. And he volunteers to be "assessed" as part of the geriatric assessment lecture within the geriatric elective each semester it is offered. He scored a perfect 30 on the MMSE the first time he took it. But he did not do as well on the Medi-Cog,[1] an assessment to measure an individual's ability to fill a pillbox. And he matter-of-factly explained the reason for this to the students during class: "Well, if I ever take enough pills to put in a pillbox, then I'll definitely ask for help filling it."

But we, my students and I, have learned other, more important lessons from Mr. M, and clearly, it's not only about his drug regimen. We have learned how to age successfully. We have learned the importance of finding a purpose and of having a reason to get up every day. We have learned the value of a social network—and its existence in many forms beyond Facebook. But more importantly, Mr. M, still wearing his familiar flannel shirt and cardigan, now has a face that lights up like a birthday cake (with 91 candles) whenever we are with him. Students, for their part, are often found practicing tai chi with Mr. M and the other residents, having lunch with them, answering questions about new medications or a newly diagnosed condition, or showing the residents how to use Skype with their grandchildren. The exchange of ideas and the other types of communicative encounters make the residents feel young and allow the students to appreciate an entire population that has been unknown to them until now, especially in this way. And although this is not to minimize the needs of the frail elderly, it does offer another side to aging, a side that many pharmacy students never encounter while in pharmacy school: not bad for an 88-year-old freshman.

1. Anderson K, Jue SG, Madaras-Kelly KJ. Identifying patients at risk for medication misman-agement: Using cognitive screens to predict a patient's accuracy in filling a pillbox. Consult Pharm 2008;23:459–72.

Truth in Action

Altruism and Justice in Pharmaceutical Care

I say that justice is truth in action.

Benjamin Disraeli

Charity is no substitute for justice withheld.

Augustine

The Power of Positivity

Jon P. Wietholter, Pharm.D., BCPS
Educator/Preceptor

As a student at the University of Pittsburgh, I was the kid that sat at the back of the classroom; the kid that did crossword puzzles and Sudoku puzzles instead of fully immersing myself in lectures; the kid that occasionally nodded off during class, dreaming of the big payday upon completion of pharmacy school. I was not going to teach. I had absolutely no interest in it. I was not going to deal with students like myself. What possible benefits were there to teaching? Less money, spoiled students (not that different from myself), and...well, let's be honest, a lot less money. And then, in a brief 2-week period on the other side of the world, everything changed.

Upon graduation in 2007, I was lucky enough to be invited to travel to South Africa as a member of the International Scholar Laureate Program's Delegation on Medicine. The experience was designed to allow students in the medical professions the opportunity to learn about a different culture and a different style of health care system. Many took the opportunity as a vacation, and I was absolutely guilty of this decision. Who wouldn't want to spend 2 weeks in a foreign land after graduation? Who wouldn't want to finish their schooling with a safari? However, others went into the experience looking at it as an opportunity to reshape themselves, and fortunately for me, I converted to this viewpoint. The experience touched me to the core, and in the end, it changed me and what it was that I stood for. It changed the way I viewed my place in the profession of pharmacy. It changed everything.

Although I was not able to provide direct medical care to patients during my experience, I was able to observe many aspects of the South African system available to them. Public and private hospitals and primary care clinics were visited, and one truth was evident throughout: adequate health care was hard to come by for the impoverished of the community. It was there, just not very accessible. One patient we encountered had been waiting for 8 hours to receive her chemotherapy.

You see, it was first-come, first-served, so waiting was her lifeline to receive needed medications. It was absurdly eye opening. To see people living in such desolate poverty and fighting for their health care made me think about the American patient complaining about a $4 prescription with a pack of cigarettes in the other hand. It made me think about the American patient that leaves against medical advice. Although I'm sure these scenarios take place in many different countries and cultures around the world, I have trouble seeing many South Africans acting in this manner. Most of the people I encountered in South Africa would plead for an opportunity to be seen and treated the way we all should be treated. And yet they were happy.

Throughout my 2 weeks in South Africa, I experienced unconscionable poverty, with literally millions of people living in thrown-together shacks. Mangled pieces of tin and scrap metal were shaped to serve as a barrier against the elements. Thousands were crammed into an area comparable to the Northwest Ohio family farms I grew up surrounded by. Two women we encountered proudly showed us their "shack" in Soweto. They beamed while we looked through a roughly 8 ft × 8 ft space that sheltered them and the rest of their family. They gleamed with pride over their ability to survive and flourish amid an evident economic disadvantage. Despite the poverty and overwhelming illness surrounding them, they were joyful. Their attitude toward material possessions was so much of a "who cares" way of thinking that I had trouble comprehending how those possessions could be a source of pride. But they definitely appeared to be proud. On deeper reflection, however, it became obvious to me that the possessions weren't what created their happiness. Their joy was derived from the relationships they had forged with neighbors, friends, and families. The relationships and circumstances that allowed them to gather what little they owned brought them joy. Their culture did not center on material possessions; it centered on the ability to enjoy what they had, not what they wanted. It was a refreshing change from what I had grown accustomed to, and that aspect of their culture continued to change me.

They're really, honestly, happy. I had never seen a culture that takes so much pride in so little. But they're truly happy. And that happiness was contagious. I found myself falling in love with a country and culture that I hadn't known anything about before my departure. I loved the beauty of the countryside, the beauty of the coastline, and, most of all, the beauty of the people. To see true happiness with what life had dealt them made me examine the way I felt about myself and the world of pharmacy. I found myself contemplating the reality that money does not reside in the same realm of importance as true happiness. The feeling of watching people smile and not worrying about whether or not their Land Rover makes them seem successful to their peers swept over me, and it made me deeply consider what my future role in the profession of pharmacy should be. I wanted others to have an experience similar to mine. I wanted others to realize that the thing that truly makes us successful is understanding what brings us joy in life. The next step was figuring out how to accomplish this, and in South Africa, half a world away, it dawned on me: I was going to teach.

What other career option could allow me the opportunity to affect both students in the United States and a culture on the other side of the world? By getting involved in the education of future pharmacists, I could hopefully instill the desire to help others, do something a little "outside the box," and aid in the care of those that need aid the most. Hopefully, students with a similar experience can build on what they learn and find a way to benefit their own personal happiness. Ideally, they will also find their niche in how to positively change a culture through their actions and efforts. Never in a million years would I have believed that I would be teaching and that it would be directly because of an experience in South Africa. But true happiness doesn't abide by the time constraints we put on our lives, and I now have trouble contemplating the times when I was not considering a career in teaching.

After accepting my current position with West Virginia University, I made it a priority to develop a fourth-year pharmacy practice rotation in South Africa so that students could experience the joyful culture that changed me. I wanted their eyes to open to the role we can play as health care providers in creating a sense of happiness and contentment with whatever life throws at us. We all should be able to look around us and say that we are truly happy with what we are doing. We should be able to feel a sense of pride in how we carry ourselves throughout our professional lives. Our focus on what is actually important in this world can change, and incorporating those changes can positively affect patient care by showing that everyone has the capability to love and be loved. No matter what trials and tribulations are put in our way, we have the opportunity to change people by how we act and deliver patient care. Every patient should be greeted with a smile because the power of a smile is that not only can it change a perception, but also a mood, an outlook on life, a way of life. Through how we practice the profession of pharmacy, we can make a difference by showing our patients that we actually do care. They should never be a number to us. They should all be treated equally despite their backgrounds, ethnicities, and any other differences that may exist. People can change and people can change you, and this simple reality should always be at the center of our focus as health care professionals. Unfortunately, this is easier said than done. Not everyone can have an experience like my trip to South Africa. However, a continuation of the international fourth-year rotation will allow more people to experience the same joyful culture that I encountered.

As a student, I was the kid that did crossword puzzles and occasionally nodded off during class. I had absolutely no desire to teach. But people do change. I changed. My professional priorities were radically rearranged, and I can attribute this conversion to my experience in South Africa. Seeing a culture that is inherently positive despite the many negatives experienced by the majority of the population on a daily basis gives me hope. Through teaching, maybe I can play a small part in bringing this concept to the generation of students now gracing our hallways. The power of positivity is immeasurable. And if I continue to follow this approach, I feel I will be truly successful as I traverse my pharmacy career. If I continue on this journey, realizing that my career path should not be about me but always about them, I will sit down at the end of the day and be truly proud of what I have accomplished. How we attempt to leave our footprint on the profession of pharmacy is solely up to us. And for me, the answer was to teach.

The Little Things
(Les Petites Choses, Las Pequeñas Cosas)

Doreen Pon, Pharm.D., BCOP
Educator

"Blanc, blanc, blanc!"

Foreigners (all foreigners are apparently "white") are a rare sight in this rural corner of Haiti, and I was attracting a lot of attention, walking down the muddy road that runs through Petite Riviere de Nippes. Although only 40 miles from the bustling city of Port-au-Prince, Petite Riviere de Nippes is a sparsely populated coastal town without electricity and running water (except when the water runs down from the mountains to the ocean after a rainstorm). Most of the inhabitants live in one-room cinderblock houses and tend a few scrawny chickens and goats in their yards. Six months after a devastating earthquake hit Haiti, the poorest country in the Western Hemisphere, I was here, along with a small team of physicians and optometrists, hoping to save a few lives by volunteering in a medical clinic.

In the absence of television, it appeared I was the only show in town today. My destination was the local daily outdoor market, where women from the surrounding countryside would bring tubs of cassavas, watermelons, and mangoes to sell. I thought I would be able to discreetly observe the locals as they went about their shopping, try to eavesdrop, and get a handle on the cadence of spoken Haitian Creole, but I was mistaken. Twenty pairs of eyes stared at me as I picked my way through the potholes. Then, 20 new sets of eyeballs locked onto me and drilled into my back as I made my way down the next stretch of road. I tried to smile, wave, and look friendly, even throwing out the occasional cheery *"Bonjour!"*, but my presence still seemed to alarm the small children playing in their yards, sending them yelling *"Blanc!"* at the top of their lungs and running for cover inside their houses. Some of the mothers started to do the same, excitedly waving their arms and shouting at their children to get inside the house as the *blanc* walked by. Growing up as a racial minority in the United States, I had experienced a fair amount of discrimination—name-calling and staring being the most obvious—but nothing had prepared me for the sad isolation I felt walking among these Haitian people I so desperately wanted to help. The villagers seemed unwelcoming and suspicious of my presence. My pre-trip vision of being welcomed into people's homes to share a watermelon and have a chubby baby thrust into my lap quickly faded from my overly vivid imagination.

Our group's first attempt to set up a mobile treatment clinic didn't go as smoothly as I would have wanted. We were disorganized and overwhelmed by the hundreds of patients who were already waiting for us when we arrived. Patients appeared confused by many of the questions we were asking during physical examinations. The multiple translations were slowing things down even more. At some point, we had to turn away more than half of the patients who had been waiting all day. Because none of us could speak Creole, we relied on our translators to apologize for the wait and explain that we were not equipped to see all the patients who had shown up that day. The crowd became angry. They had had nothing to eat or drink all day, and now, they were being told to go home, without being examined by one of the doctors. One of the women complained of a headache from standing in the sun. She demanded that I give her a pain medication so that she could at least walk back home. I could only hand her a tablet of acetaminophen, without being able to express my apologies for her wait. I was supposed to be here to help, and yet I felt like a complete failure.

On a sunny Sunday morning, we held a special optometry clinic. There weren't too many pharmacy needs today, so I took a seat outside with the patients. I had been in Haiti for a week now and could manage three phrases in Haitian Creole and a few muddled words in French. Two older women in their Sunday dresses approached me. I managed to get past my name, where I was from, and how old I was. Then, they started asking me something about my mother and father. I was perplexed. One of them motioned like she was rocking a baby in her arms. I made a pouty face and shook my head. No. No baby. Then, they repeated something about my mother and father and covered their hearts with their hands and pointed to the sky. Did I love my parents? Were my parents in heaven? Why weren't my parents with me? I felt like the village idiot. Even if I could figure out what they were asking, my language skills didn't extend beyond numbers and single words. A neatly groomed man appeared by my side. He asked me a question in French, which I accidentally answered half in French and half in Spanish. "¿Habla español?"

My rescuer! We had found a common language. He interrogated me to satisfy the curiosity of the growing crowd of people around us. Were my parents living? Did I live with them? Why weren't they with me? Did I have a husband? How many brothers and sisters? Cousins? Family, obviously, was very important to Haitians. A few of the young girls put their arms next to mine. My skin was so pale! They shyly touched my arm and then stroked their own arms, comparing the texture. What was my name? I wrote it out for them and pronounced it slowly. They giggled and asked for my pen so that they could write their names for me. Then, they pronounced their names slowly, enunciating each syllable, just as I had done. Suddenly, everyone was around me, waiting to write their names in my notebook and introduce themselves. Could I take a few photos of my new friends? The young girls nodded enthusiastically, hit poses like fashion models, and then quickly dashed back to my camera to see how their photos came out. Soon, even the old women were being pushed in front of the camera and coached on how to pose.

When the crowd finally thinned out, my Spanish-speaking rescuer explained that he was a schoolteacher and that he was very happy to have been able to get some eyedrops to help with his chronic eye irritation. He carefully pulled two little green bottles of artificial tears out of his pants pocket to show me.

"We are very poor, very poor. We need groups like this to help the people here. How long do you stay? When do you come back? You will write to me, yes? Don't forget your friends here in Haiti!" he said, earnestly.

It was the simplest of things—artificial tears—nothing heroic, nothing lifesaving, nothing to write home about. And yet, it was the most rewarding experience of my trip. For a moment, I was able to view the work that we were trying to do in that little village from the perspective of a villager, rather than from my own lofty, idealistic perspective. Maybe it really is the little things in life that make a difference.

Muy Amable (Too Kind)

Sally A. Arif, Pharm.D., BCPS
Educator

" You are too kind"—that's what the elderly, 4'6" Mayan woman said to me in her broken Spanish after waiting more than 20 minutes for something to relieve her arthritic pain. She had no sense of urgency or annoyance in her voice, only appreciation. Her dark, wrinkled, thin face had seen many long days in the sun. It took her a couple of minutes to feel for my hand to give it a tight squeeze, as her untreated cataracts had severely diminished her vision. I realized that the pair of sunglasses and the few tablets of acetaminophen we gave her were more than she had anticipated from our medical staff's visit to her small Guatemalan village. I felt an overwhelming sense of value, sympathy, and pity for her. How was it that such simple medical attention could engender so much gratitude in her? Her lack of a sense of entitlement was humbling. She slowly rose and made her way up the dirt road. She would arrive hours later at her small shanty, where she would continue to make hundreds of tortillas until she could not longer stand the pain in her wrists.

Waking up to the sound of roosters and construction at 6:00 each morning, only to be met with a bone-chilling cold shower and simple breakfast of beans, was not what motivated us. Nor was our motivation the 1-mile walk up the unpaved, dusty road as we breathed in the polluted smog that filled the morning air. Rather, it was the first glimpse of the lines of patients awaiting our arrival outside the makeshift free clinic each day that motivated us. Seeing those patients' anxious faces was what gave us the first jolt of energy. We realized that today was not just another clinic day—it was another day to make a difference in hundreds of lives. Although each 12-hour workday would leave our bodies tired and aching, it would leave our souls soaring with a sense of satisfaction because we knew that our patients had received the care they desperately needed.

During our clinical careers, many of us in the health care field subconsciously create an emotional barrier to separate us from our patients. With the evolution of medications and medical devices, we rely on drugs or tests to give us many answers. In Guatemala, there were no catheterization labs, OR suites, MRI machines, or dialysis machines at our disposal. There were only exam rooms separated by bedsheets and a pharmacy made up of five large suitcases filled with analgesics, antimicrobials, vitamins, GI agents, and antihistamines. These suitcases accompanied us from village to village, where we built our open-air clinics in schools, churches, community centers, and any other space we could find. Our clinic in the village of San Martin was in the parking lot of an elementary school. The open suitcases that held our medications sat on the hot concrete ground adjacent to 40 parked motorcycles and bikes. We were lucky to find an old rickety table to use as our dispensing area. While we prepared their medications, the patients would share their remarkable life stories. Maria, a small 5-year-old girl, was seen by our pediatricians for trouble breathing. We could hear her wheezing as she cautiously approached our table. The pediatrician documented newly diagnosed asthma and her need for an albuterol inhaler on her triage paperwork. Maria's mother described cooking in her poorly ventilated kitchen and her daughter's long walk to the local school through the dust- and smoke-filled air as the cause of her daughter's problems. We quickly realized that without the use of a spacer, Maria would have difficulty receiving her entire dose with each inhalation. Through creative thinking, we used a small Styrofoam cup with a hole cut in the bottom to place the mouthpiece through, thus making our own spacer. After demonstrating how to use the inhaler and spacer, we watched as Maria mastered the technique. This type of interaction drove home the basics of patient care. This raw experience allowed our team to recognize that all the bells and whistles of modern medicine can never replace the fundamental skills of listening, connecting with our patients, and being creative.

In Guatemala, our role as pharmacists was in many ways similar to what we do day to day in the States. We still had to decipher unintelligible handwriting and decide, based on our limited formulary, the best therapeutic option for each patient. With the local diet consisting of black coffee and spicy foods, GI upset was a common complaint.

We often gave out proton pump inhibitors or over-the-counter antacids until we quickly ran out of our donated supply. Aside from the scarce resources, the main difference was the need to break through the language and cultural barriers to provide the best counseling. Jose, a 12-year-old boy who attended a local junior high, arrived at the clinic with his father, who spoke only a Mayan dialect called K'iche'. Our reliance on Jose as our only translator from K'iche' to Spanish became evident as we evaluated the source of his father's shoulder pain. We were also forced to work off of many assumptions. With our elderly patients, we asked ourselves, "Does this person have normal renal or hepatic function?" With young mothers receiving antibiotic suspensions for their young children with otitis media, we asked ourselves, "Would these mothers have proper refrigeration to store the medication we give them?" Although our aim was always to "do no harm," without the proper follow-up, we could never be entirely sure of the end result of our work.

My desire to be a lifelong learner, as well as my role as an educator, inspires me to go on medical missions. However, I realized that my role as a preceptor on an international medical mission allowed my students to experience patient-centered care in its purest form. In the open-air makeshift pharmacy set up in the parking lot of a community center, our patients waited unwearyingly on the white lawn chairs we had set up earlier that day. They would watch as we poured a 30- to 60-day supply of their medication into Ziploc bags marked with their name and basic instructions for use in Spanish. I saw patients not only verbalize their gratitude, but also physically reach out to hug and even kiss the pharmacy student who educated them about their disease and medications. There were no complaints about insurance co-pays or lines of impatiently waiting patients; nor was there any lack of desire to be counseled about directions and side effects. As a teacher, I was overjoyed because the clinical lessons presented themselves effortlessly. Students were afforded the opportunity to apply their skills such as compounding. This was true in a pediatric case in which the students were challenged to make a ketoconazole suspension using 200-mg tablets and mineral oil for a baby with a severe case of tinea capitis on her scalp. After calculating the proper concentration, one student used a Ziploc bag containing the proper amount of tablets and a rock as her makeshift mortar and pestle. I watched as the pharmacy student sat on the curb next to the baby's mother, showing her how to precisely draw up the correct daily dose. The counseling session ended with the mother putting the baby and medication in the sling around her back and giving the student a warm embrace. We could not deny that the hours spent counseling patients left our mouths dry and that administering vaccinations to the young and old left our hands tired. But, knowing we had provided much-needed health care to the underserved left us filled with a sense of value.

The pictures we took during this short 2-week trip show patients smiling after a visit to our clinic, our medical staff bonding with the local people through a game of soccer after a long clinic day, and the beautiful, lush landscape of Guatemala. When one of the patients claimed to me, on the last day of clinic, that the glasses we gave her "opened up a whole new world," I could only think, these people, this experience have done the same for me. We had all realized that the value of our experience in Guatemala not only allowed us to grow as practitioners, but also as humanitarians.

Uko na Uwezo (You Have the Power)

Joy Vongspanich, Pharm.D.
Resident

After a 1-hour-long bumpy journey down a winding dirt road in Western Kenya, my colleagues and I finally arrive in the rural village of Nasianda. Welcoming us are the smiling faces of the local women and men. Their outstretched hands are ready to greet us with warm and unique Kenyan handshakes. The children are hiding behind one another—fearful, yet terribly curious about the *muzungu* who have come to their village. Standing under the shade of an avocado tree, I look around and see them watching us; they appear grateful that we have come to bring knowledge and excited to see what we have to share. Taking in the fresh country air, I walk past the roaming chickens, the children who think they cannot be seen, and the wandering kittens, toward the communal mud hut. Entering the hut, my eyes slowly adjust from the blinding brightness of the sun outside to the contrasting shadows of the hut. It is furnished with a few wooden chairs, benches, and coffee tables all covered with a tin roof, delicately permitting small bursts of sunlight into the room.

Here, my colleagues and I set up for the first of a four-class series on HIV education. Waiting for the lesson to begin, a group of high school boys, young mothers, men, and a village grandmother sit with class-provided manuals in hand. On the hard wooden benches and chairs in this stifling hut, everyone patiently waits for class to begin, yet clearly eager to learn. We discuss in detail the specifics of HIV transmission, prevention, the disease course, and the cultural beliefs and practices that significantly contribute to the spread of this deadly virus. This class of adults is more than attentive, soaking up every bit of information provided. We have lively discussions between the men and women in which voices are finally heard, and ideas and disbeliefs are hopefully clarified. Myths are spoken aloud and dispelled.

During the hours and days spent in Nasianda, I begin to feel an ease with our presence wash over the town. The children slowly become more courageous and greet us, venturing into the areas that we, the *muzungu*, are in. Still, moral standards and local standing continue to influence the class, including what is said and accepted as truth. The myths spoken by a boy are more easily dispelled than the words spoken by the village pastor. As difficult and frustrating as it is to hear the customs that inevitably lead to the spread of HIV such as spouse inheritance, extramarital sex to have children, and traditional healers, it is harder still when evidence-based knowledge falls on ears that are closed to alternatives. In working to combat the spread of a virus that has already claimed more than 7 percent of the population, these disbeliefs must be overcome if this trip to Kenya is to have an impact. Thus, the ease and trust gained during the hours we spend in Nasianda are accompanied by a sense of hesitation and disquiet.

Because the local pastor is a strictly religious man, condoms are not part of his lifestyle or a tool he is comfortable counseling his parishioners about. However, after many involved conversations, he learns of the reality of the world and of the conflicts in his preaching that may affect the safety of his congregation and community. Although my colleagues and I are not trying to change anyone's religious beliefs or morals, if compromises can be made to help many, our duty is to make them happen, such as with this pastor and the use of condoms. Gradually, the local pastor begins to bend in his thinking, and the class members similarly become more accepting of the facts we teach them. Indeed, by the end of our ninth hour, a balance appears to be struck between the pastor and the class.

With more modern teachings provided to the local people from respected community members and the information we are sharing, it is hoped that the local villagers receive the message of prevention and understand that they are empowered to take control of their own health. By providing information, allowing voices to be heard, answering questions, and proving myths false, the hope is that each person will leave the class empowered—that each will start taking responsibility for his or her own health, knowing that no one else can or will. It is amazing, as an outsider, to see the transformation brought about by knowledge.

It is easy to forget that, aside from pharmacy's clinical interventions, there are many other ways in which pharmacists can help change the world. Our knowledge of medications, diseases, and pertinent counseling points can have great power to help others. In situations such as this, in which HIV/AIDS is viewed as a death sentence and treatment is not always possible, education is invaluable. It is easy to focus on the medical treatments for diseases because this is what health care professionals such as pharmacists have been trained in and know. It is more difficult for us to remember that, for diseases with no cure, in areas where distributive justice may not exist, and where standard of care correlates with resources and not evidence, it is education that will save lives.

When There Is No Guardian

Lauren J. Jonkman, Pharm.D., BCPS
Clinician/Educator

S he was the first woman that I ever saw die. I will never forget her face, or the chain of events surrounding her death.

I went to Africa to work with a physician friend in a government hospital in a fairly large capital city. My friend had already been there for a month, working on the women's infectious diseases ward. I came to the country and the hospital as a pharmacist to learn more about how medicine is practiced in a limited-resource setting and to help her and the rest of her team in whatever way I could.

As a clinician, I feel most comfortable working in free clinics and community health centers, and in fact, I prefer to work in settings with limited resources. I pride myself on my ability to provide effective, evidence-based care without all the high-end, expensive, often unnecessary "bells and whistles" associated with much of the care provided in our American health system. I relish the challenge of making do with only what's truly necessary and helping my patients understand that they really don't *need* that new medication they saw advertised on television, nor do they *need* to go to the emergency room when they wake up with a sore throat. There are safer, more efficient, more cost-effective solutions to their problems.

I knew that I was going to a poor country—its GDP was under $800 per person per year—and I knew that I would see poverty and suffering that was intensely different from the poverty and suffering at home. Given my experience working in low-resource settings, though, I thought I was prepared to practice as a clinical pharmacist in this and any setting. Although I understood that the constraints on resources would be much greater there than at home, I naively underestimated the differences between these two countries.

When I first arrived, I was very focused on the apparent injustice I observed when working within the constraints of the government formulary. It was archaic and barely seemed to meet the needs of the population. My frustration would escalate when I realized that the only available ACE inhibitor was captopril. Really? Captopril? Wouldn't a once-daily option cost the same? Similarly, I would become exasperated trying to manage patients with insulin-dependent diabetes at the hospital's weekly diabetes clinic with one "random" fasting blood glucose every 3 months and only regular insulin and lente. Lente? When was the last time I used or even saw lente? Who uses lente?! But then, I started to realize that access to an appropriate formulary was not at all the most pressing issue.

The hospital, built decades earlier, bore little similarity to hospitals in the United States. The main building, five stories high, was built around a large central courtyard. Although natural sunlight streams through this central opening, illuminating the balconies/hallways, little light actually reaches the overcrowded patient rooms. And even though hospital staff diligently mop the floors more frequently than at home, the hospital still had a dingy, unloved, forgotten-about feeling.

The free medical ward was divided in two—the right side for men and the left for women. Patient rooms, which, in the United States, would only fit two beds, contained as many as 12 beds with almost no privacy (though a sheet *could* be drawn around for a private exam). The women's side of the medicine ward was further divided into communicable and noncommunicable disease rooms—we worked with patients in the former.

Although the hospital is considered a 500-bed hospital, rarely would there be so few patients. When the census would rise, overflow patients would be placed first in beds and then on just mattresses on the open verandah, attached to the outside of the hospital. I was in the country in May, just as the rainy season was ending. The days could get stifling hot, but the temperature at night often dropped into the low 50s. Essentially, overflow patients were relegated to sleeping outside, no matter what the weather.

The patient who taught me the most…"she"…was admitted to the ward during the second week of my experience in the hospital. All patients are expected to bring a guardian to help feed, bathe, clothe, and care for them while they are ill. The guardian is by that patient's side 24 hours a day, except when cooking meals and laundering clothes, often sleeping under the patient's bed at night. But guardians also serve another very important, essential role—they advocate for their loved one, making sure that they are seen every day by a physician, that they receive the medicines prescribed, and that they receive any blood work and testing necessary—guardians even track down wheelchairs to bring their family members to radiology for chest x-rays. And, if the patient dies, their guardian wails over them, weeping for their lost life.

This patient was without a guardian and was assigned a bed on the verandah. While our team covered the back two rooms on the ward, another expat physician was responsible for patients in the first room and on the verandah. We noticed after the first few days that the other physician did not seem to round on all the patients on the verandah every day, so we started to see the missed patients on days when we had time.

When we first saw her, we were not sure what was wrong, not an uncommon occurrence in this setting with little diagnostic capabilities and even more limited treatment modalities. She was about 30 years old, HIV positive, but she was already on antiretrovirals (ARVs). She was febrile and had some gastrointestinal upset but otherwise seemed well. Because of the limited diagnostic capabilities, she was started on a typical cocktail of broad-spectrum antibiotics and antimalarials and seemed to be improving.

However, one afternoon, we were hurried to her side by another patient's guardian. She had fallen off the bed and was bleeding from where her IV tubing had pulled out. She was barely responsive and was unable to answer any questions about what had happened. However, with a desperate look in her eyes, she envisaged her death and and told us she was terrified that she would never see her daughter again. No one on the verandah was able to provide us with any more history. She was febrile and hypotensive, but why? Sepsis? Pulmonary embolism? We were still unsure what ultimately was wrong with her.

I rushed to the supply room to get another bag of IV fluids and more blankets to help prop her up. As I watched the team by her side, working to stabilize her, I stood back, feeling entirely helpless, barely noticing the nurse who tsked at the waste of so many clean blankets. Surely the nurse's indifference was a symptom of the chronic lack of resources in a setting of unbelievably high mortality, not of her true feelings and values.

Soon, our patient was moved off the verandah and into the "high dependency unit," less to provide more intensive care, as there was little more that could be done, and more to calm other patients and guardians. At this point, with such limited space and an ample team, I stood back and took in the scene, unsure of how else to help. I could see the look of panic in her eyes—she knew she was dying—and we were unable to stop it. Worse, she was surrounded by *mzungus* (foreigners) who couldn't even speak her language. It was painful standing there, feeling so incapable and inadequate in her last moments, unable to provide her with the comfort she most needed. And in the end, she had no one to wail for her. Where was her dignity in death?

I felt utterly defeated that afternoon on the 3-mile walk back to our home. I felt entirely responsible for her death. I should have noticed that she was still on the verandah, alone. I should have noticed that her clinical situation was worsening. I should have been there to make sure she got the care she needed. These ideas kept filtering through my mind. I kept asking myself, "Why did she die?" Was it because she didn't have a guardian? Was it because her bed was on the verandah, far enough away from other guardians and staff, who could have watched over her and advocated for her a little more?

Maybe it was because the system has so few resources that everything seems to be falling apart? In this and many other low-income countries in Africa, health care providers are dying faster than their patients from HIV, and those who aren't dying are actively being recruited to careers in other, wealthier countries, and can you blame them? I can't imagine working in a system where medication stock-outs are commonplace, reagents for basic laboratory tests are often unavailable, and most diagnostic technologies are simply out of reach—where patients die and you never even know why. Without an organized system for patient hand-offs, it's no wonder that patients get left on the porch for days without being seen. Billions of dollars are being spent to ensure that she had access to ARVs, but so little funding is allocated to shore up a health care infrastructure that is woefully outdated; doing so could have prevented not only her death, but also an untold number of other unnecessary deaths.

The frustrations surrounding her death hit me in a way that is difficult to describe. Ultimately, she died because she was a woman, because she was African, and because she was poor. She had no voice, no one to speak up for her, no one to fight her battles. She was guardian-less in many ways.

When people ask me about my experiences "in Africa," it's difficult to describe exactly what I was witness to in a meaningful way. When I first returned home, I was exceedingly pessimistic. What hope is there for this system to change? Is it just luck when patients get better, or lack of luck when they don't? What is our role in changing this system? How can I get frustrated with the mundane issues of access and inequity at home, considering the exponentially greater injustice I witnessed? I had grossly underestimated all the resources we truly have in the United States, even in what are considered "limited-resource" settings. When patients and other health care providers would ask me about medical services that were essentially unnecessary, I would look at them incredulously. I would be struck by their requests, but how could they know that in other parts of the world, people are dying for lack of basic medical services or even more fundamental human needs.

After 3 years, I've come to take a slightly different view. I'm more forward with my physician colleagues when I see resources being wasted, and I have regular talks with my patients about evidence-based care and the truth about "rationing." I am again able to see the impact of resource limitations on my patients at home. We should get upset when we see injustice, regardless of where we see it. I know that my role, as a pharmacist, is often viewed as very drug-centric, but I know that my role is greater. As a pharmacist, patient care provider, and citizen, I must be there to advocate for my patients—both in a local sense and in a global one. They need for me to be their voice when no one else will hear them, and I will never forget the woman who taught me this lesson.

Good Intentions Are Not Enough

Learning from Our Mistakes

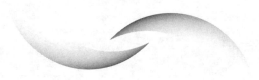

Finite to fail, but infinite to venture.

Emily Dickinson

*Once we realize that imperfect under-
standing is the human condition there is no
shame in being wrong, only in failing to correct our mistakes.*

George Soros

Diary of a Wimpy Pharmacist

Doreen Pon, Pharm.D., BCOP
Educator

People tell me that working in oncology must be tough because it's so depressing. I usually mumble that it isn't really as depressing as they might think. They seem to get a little squinty, suspicious look in their eyes. I know they're thinking I must be a cold-hearted, motherless freak of nature. I want to explain that I wasn't always like this. I, too, used to be like them—wimpy and afraid to talk about death.

When meeting my oncology patients for the first time, my ice-breaker topics usually revolved around food, family, or travel—topics that would generally get the shy patients to talk and lighten the mood of the depressed ones. Evelyn Wong was in her 40s and in the hospital with newly diagnosed acute myelogenous leukemia. Leukemia patients would generally be facing a long hospitalization and frequent readmissions, so usually, I would try to find out a little about them so that I could at least match a name with a face. I happened to walk into Evelyn's room as she was contemplating the contents of her breakfast tray with some disgust. She picked up her entire egg omelet with a plastic fork and held it toward me.

"Would you eat this? It looks like insulation material!"

I laughed and told her that the hospital didn't take a very friendly stance on any living life forms being present on food trays. She let out a heavy sigh and said that the thing she missed the most was a salad. A produce fan myself, I told her about some delicious grape tomatoes I had picked up at the local supermarket. I could tell she was disappointed in my low standards for tomatoes.

"Nothing beats tomatoes from the farmers' market!" she exclaimed.

From then on, whenever she was readmitted, we would catch up on our latest food finds. I came to find out that she had a college-aged son who played the guitar and was in a band. She glowed with pride whenever she talked about him. I eventually inquired about her Chinese-sounding last name. It was her first husband's last name, she revealed.

Her current husband didn't seem to be very supportive. I never saw him visit her during any of her admissions, and she rarely talked about him. It made me sad. She was such a sweet lady and didn't deserve to battle her disease by herself.

Evelyn eventually completed all of her cycles of chemotherapy, and I didn't see her for a year. Then I got a message from her on my voice mail. What did I know about this monoclonal antibody drug for leukemia? Her leukemia was back, and her physician had recommended that she be treated with this drug, but she was worried about the side effects and whether the drug would work for her.

Honestly, the practical, evidence-based side of me wasn't very hopeful. Her type of leukemia carried a poor prognosis, and response rates with the drug weren't all that impressive. But I called her back and told her that while the drug appeared to benefit only a small number of patients, one couldn't predict which patients would respond. I tried to reassure her that the side effect profile of the drug was different from that of traditional chemotherapy, so she might find it easier to tolerate. When I hung up, I felt like I had lied to her and let her down. Was she asking for my honest personal opinion, or did she just want to reassure herself that she had made the right decision? Even if I could have figured out whether she wanted an honest opinion, I wouldn't have had the courage to tell her that my guts were telling me that her odds didn't look good.

She was admitted to the hospital to receive her treatment. She seemed more frightened and less optimistic this time. She said she wasn't really scared of dying, but the thought of not being able to see her son get married and have a family really made her sad. I could feel a waterfall of tears starting to build up behind my eyeballs and willed myself to keep it together. Most patients don't really want pity. They just want someone who listens to them. I gave her a hug and told her that her son knew that she loved him.

Eventually, Evelyn was admitted for the last time. I knew that she wasn't doing well and that she probably wouldn't make it out of the hospital this time, but I wasn't prepared for how bad she looked. I guess I never really noticed how tiny she was because her sunny personality usually made me overlook her size. But now, she looked so frail, lying in bed, unable to speak, her lips black and crusted over with dried blood. She greeted me with a limp lift of her hand. The chemotherapy had destroyed most of the cells of her blood, and she was having a hard time recovering from the neutropenia, anemia, and thrombocytopenia. I suggested some medications that could be applied to her oral mucosa to help control the bleeding and avoided going into her room to check on her after that. I felt like I had let her down by emphasizing the positive benefits of her chemotherapy and neglecting to fully inform her about all the side effects she might experience or telling her that the treatment might even kill her. I didn't have any therapies to offer her and didn't really know what to say to her. I broke my own cardinal rule of being there to listen to my patients. I was a wimpy pharmacist.

I was working on the day Evelyn died. Her son had stayed overnight in her room with her. I thought about going up to him and telling him what a neat person his mom had been and how much she loved talking about him, but I didn't really know him, and I felt I would be intruding on his privacy. And maybe I also felt some guilt for encouraging his mother to pursue what turned out to be her final therapy. I regret that I never said anything to him, because I think Evelyn would have appreciated it.

Over the years, I've crossed paths with more patients like Evelyn—patients who have touched me and inspired me with their strength, gracious optimism, and absolute lack of self-pity. Each one has made me a little stronger, a little more prepared to offer support in the face of bad news, a little less wimpy.

Richard Ryban was a jokester. He was, of course, completely bald from his chemotherapy, but that didn't keep him from walking around the hospital wearing a Dodgers baseball cap with furry gray "hair" attached and getting a kick out of watching other patients and families doing a double-take when they passed him in the halls. Every morning, he would good-naturedly pester his physician to discharge him.

"Look Doc, I'm feeling GREAT! You can kick me out today because I know there's someone just dying to sleep in this lumpy bed. And it ain't me."

Richard ended up needing an allogeneic hematopoietic stem cell transplant. When the student pharmacists and I began to counsel him about the 15 medications he would need to take after discharge, he held up his hand and pointed to his wife, telling us that she was the "boss and the brains" in the family. I quipped back that he was very lucky to have such a great "boss-lady" to take care of him.

I must have hit on Richard's soft spot, because the usually never-serious Richard started to tear-up, and his voice quivered as he told me, "Yeah, I don't deserve her. She's great."

Richard eventually ended up developing complications from his transplant and landed in the intensive care unit with respiratory distress. Over the course of 10 days, he developed progressive respiratory, renal, and hepatic failure. While the student pharmacists and I would be hanging out in the ICU, waiting for rounds to start, Richard's wife would usually poke her head out of Richard's room to say "Hi" and to ask about any changes in his therapy. At first, she was hopeful that the combination of antibiotics would pull him through, and so were we. As the days dragged on, and Richard began developing more complications, his wife's optimism turned into concern over his suffering. After a lengthy discussion with the medical team, his wife made the difficult decision to terminally extubate him.

I was determined not to be a wimp this time. I was still hesitant about intruding on someone's moment of personal sorrow, but I didn't want to feel the regret of not being there to at least acknowledge a personal loss, regardless of whether I could offer help. So I offered a hug to Richard's wife and told her how apparent it was that he loved her, how complimentary he always was when he mentioned her, and what a wonderful spirit and attitude he had. Of course, I made her cry, but I wasn't afraid of her tears. I felt sadness for her sorrow, but I didn't feel guilt. She thanked me for my kind words and for always watching over Richard's therapies, even right up to the end. It made her feel that everything that could be done was being done.

And with that, I began to conquer my wimpiness. I would not feel so guilt-ridden that I could not talk to patients whose treatments had failed. I would not be afraid to "intrude" during moments of sorrow. I would not be hesitant to talk honestly about death and dying with patients who asked. I would not be depressed by the loss of my patients. I would carefully store each loss as a reminder of the preciousness of life itself.

I think Evelyn would be proud of me.

¿Cómo se dice...?

Keri A. Sims, Pharm.D., BCPS
Clinician

When I was very young, I was quite shy. As a second-born child, I could count on my older sister (the firstborn) to speak for me whether I wanted her to or not. Once I reached high school, something changed. I realized that I had spent many years wondering why I wasn't getting the attention that I desired. It became quite obvious that people don't notice wallflowers. If you want to be heard and noticed, you have to speak up. Since then, I have become a "good communicator." At least that's what my instructors, employers, and colleagues told me throughout high school, college, and my current career. My letters of recommendation always included "strong communication skills" or "is an effective communicator." So, it was quite a shock to my system when my communication skills were stripped from me while on a mission trip in Guatemala.

I traveled with a group from the States to work with a ministry in Guatemala City that cared for the spiritual and physical needs of Guatemalans who were living and working in the city's garbage dump. To work in the garbage dump, you did not need to be educated or even old enough to be employed. In the dump, there were children who appeared to be 6 or 7 but were actually malnourished 10- or 11-year-olds and men and women who appeared to be in their 80s but were likely in their 50s, aged by years of sun, cooking over open fires in the home, alcoholism, and malnutrition. All of them sifting through piles of waste. Therefore, the only requirement for this job was despair and resilience. This was the work that nobody else wanted, rummaging through other people's garbage to collect things that had value. Cardboard, aluminum, metal, and plastics could be sold. Clothing, old kitchen utensils, or a broken frame could be used personally, and a half-eaten apple could, of course, help fill an empty stomach. Although the garbage dump was city property, many had built homes in the area surrounding the dump. They were squatters.

We had the opportunity to be part of a mobile soup kitchen that brought lunch to those working in the dump. We entered the dump at a high point and made our way down a steep decline. As we descended into the dump, the hills of garbage became mountains, and the air became more and more pungent and rancid. It was apparent that I would not be able to hold my breath for an hour, but I did tend to keep my mouth closed, fearing that I might taste the foulness of the air. We watched as men, women, and children left their stake in the garbage and raced to get in line for the little red pickup that brought lunch. We also watched as many workers did not leave their stations because they knew there was a limited supply of food and they could not afford to lose time by waiting in line and still go hungry. Vultures circled overhead. Packs of scrawny, grungy dogs and wild pigs scavenged through the garbage right beside the workers. As garbage trucks drove in, many would run to the trucks, even jump onto the back of them to get first dibs on the fresh garbage. People use the term *living hell* rather recklessly, but it is an appropriate description of what I observed.

As part of our mission trip, we visited a Lutheran grade school that educated children who, if not supported by that same ministry, would be working alongside their mothers in the garbage dump. Their uniforms and backpacks had been provided to them by the ministry. Each day after school, they left their uniform at the ministry to be laundered in fear that if the uniforms went home, they would not return, and they definitely would not be clean.

The children went home to a one-room shanty with cardboard walls, dirt floors, an old mattress, and a bucket in the corner as their only toilet. I sat among the schoolchildren as we watched some of the other children sing a song they had prepared for us. I felt uncomfortable. I wondered if the children got tired of North Americans or gringos roaming through their school. Did they feel like they were on display, as if they were animals at a zoo?

The little girl next to me has the glow and beauty of a 6-year-old child. With her clean uniform, well-groomed hair, and breakfast and lunch provided to her each day, she could be on the front of *Parents* magazine. She looks at me with her big brown eyes, and we exchange smiles.

I am very capable of saying, *"Hola. Como esta? Como se llama?"* (Hello. How are you? What's your name?), but I don't. What if she starts telling me all sorts of things that I can't understand? How do you tell a 6-year-old that you don't speak Spanish, when you just did? As we sat there, she hesitantly raised her hand and placed it on my knee. I smiled at her and put my arm around her.

It became quite clear that I was so absorbed in my own fears of rejection that I couldn't even reach out to this young girl. She was willing to take a risk by reaching out to a fair-skinned blonde woman, because despite the risk of rejection, she saw the benefit of a universal language (a hand held or a hug exchanged).

My instructors, employers, and colleagues failed to say, "She's an effective verbal communicator, but her nonverbal communication skills suck." It was obvious that when my verbal communication skills were taken away in Guatemala, I became all the more uncomfortable with nonverbal communication.

This interaction with the young girl helped me realize that so many of my patients "speak a different language." Granted, they speak English, but as inpatients on a Veterans Affairs Medical Center floor, they often speak a different dialect. Each patient's "dialect" is formed by his or her own personal experiences, struggles, desires, fears, and background. One's "dialect" may be influenced by having been in combat, another's by being homeless, and still another's by struggling with alcoholism or coping with multiple chronic diseases. I will never be able to fully understand every patient's dialect. That doesn't mean that I can't try to communicate with them. I can get over myself, venture into my uncomfortable zone, and utilize the universal language of nonverbal communication. I have the opportunity to actually show that I care by sitting beside them, holding a hand or patting a knee. In doing so, I can break down some barriers that exist in our verbal communication as well.

It took a population plagued with hopelessness and despair to teach me something that no professor ever could.

Reflections on the 2009–2010 PGY1 Residency Year

Charnicia E. Huggins, Pharm.D., M.S.
Educator

I can still wince when I think about one particular experience that occurred during my PGY1 residency. It involved an older black female patient whose total parenteral nutrition (TPN) order was delayed because I missed reading a few words—the most important words—in her medical chart: short bowel syndrome. Several physicians had visited the patient and her husband during her hospital stay, and TPN had been recommended for her. Since adult TPN orders were almost exclusively written by clinical pharmacists or pharmacy residents, I, as the pharmacy resident on-call at that time, was the last roadblock to her receiving this essential nutrition.

Nutrition evaluations seemed long and tedious to me, most likely because I was not yet comfortable doing them. I was post-call when I finally got around to the patient. I had visited the room earlier and spoke with the patient and her husband. I knew that they were well aware of her deteriorating clinical condition and had been informed that she was in dire need of TPN. They sounded so desperate, and so confident that this was what she needed, and I badly wanted to help...but I also wanted to be sure that I was doing the right thing. I knew I had to read the notes in her medical chart. That was obvious. But how to distinguish between a patient's need for TPN, per the assumptions of an adamant physician, and a patient's actual need, based on the medical evidence provided—that was not so simple. I needed to make a decision based on evidence-based medicine, not based on my sympathy for the patient. I had to digest everything and write a note in the patient's chart. Because I was not yet confident in this area—nutrition support pharmacy—I waited until the morning so that I would not have to make the decision independently. However, I was on-call the night before, so waiting until morning pushed me into post-call hours.

I contacted my preceptor, who told me I could delegate the patient to the incoming on-call resident, but I was determined to complete the assignment myself. I reviewed the patient with my preceptor and detailed, or so I thought, her medical history, her labs, and other pertinent information. I even remember revisiting the patient's chart more than once to answer a question posed by my preceptor. Despite this back and forth work, I still managed to overlook that one key phrase, the crux of the TPN request. Based on the information provided to my preceptor, we decided that the patient was not yet eligible for TPN. She would instead be maintained on fluids, such as dextrose, until my preceptor performed a reevaluation on Monday morning. I wrote my note in the patient's chart and left the hospital that day thinking I had done a thorough job. Although I had ultimately denied the patient the TPN order that she so desperately requested—and needed—I had followed the rules and not been swayed by my feelings or the convincing words spoken by the patient's husband. He was not a trained medical professional, anyway; he was only parroting the words spoken to him by someone else. Still, it was not easy to erase that couple from my mind. My shift was over, but the memories remained.

When I returned to the hospital that Monday morning, I was ready to face the challenges of the day. I had gotten some much-needed rest and my next on-call shift was days away. Then the phone rang—it was the nutrition support preceptor. "Did the patient you called me about over the weekend have short bowel syndrome?" she asked. "Was it written in the patient's medical chart?" I didn't think so…that term did not sound familiar to me. I didn't even know what it was. My preceptor was convinced that the error was the physician's, not mine. She had stood up for me but just wanted to make sure that she had done the right thing. I was glad to confirm her suspicions—I knew exactly what the physician had written! And he had written exactly what he should have written. There it was in black and white: "short bowel syndrome." Yet I had overlooked it.

I have always known that I am not infallible. I make mistakes just like everyone else. I was far from an expert. But I also knew that I had failed—the patient, my preceptor, and myself. I cried that day. Maybe they were tears of regret for my procrastinating and not completing the nutrition evaluation earlier, before the weight of the stress and tiredness of the on-call shift pressed so heavily on my mind and body. Maybe it was due to my realization that I had not been as thorough as I had thought, or maybe, just maybe, it was pent-up emotion from all the experiences I had endured since the start of the residency until then. Whatever the true cause of those tears, I now can look back and see that I should have recognized my limitations, especially my post-call limitations, rather than push myself unnecessarily and at a patient's expense. Deadlines, boundaries, restrictions—they were all there for a reason. When preceptors caringly but firmly questioned why we pharmacy residents remained at the hospital after enduring our 24-hour on-call responsibilities, they were not trying to annoy us. They were looking out for us...and in doing so, they were looking out for the patients, too. I didn't think of that at the time.

Thankfully, the patient was reevaluated and TPN was started, but not by me. My note in the patient's chart will remain, as part of the patient's permanent medical record. My memory of that incident will also remain. It is a cautionary tale when I want to do just one more thing, and my body is telling me to rest. It is a reminder to take my time and do things correctly, the first time. It is a red flag, warning me that while mistakes can and do continue to occur, the same mistake should not occur repeatedly.

Thankfully, I don't have many such stories to tell.

I am not, today, where I started. I am more confident, more knowledgeable, and more competent, which is what I expected to be after completing a year of residency. Yet there is a lot more to learn, to know, to remember. The memory of that TPN patient is not one that I like to dwell on, but it remains etched in my mind, and it should. My failures, my mistakes—they are my building blocks for success. It all contributes to the person I am today and can be used as learning lessons for those who come after me.

A Passion for Practice: Perspectives from a Resident and a Preceptor

Christine K. Yocum, Pharm.D.
Resident

Seena L. Haines, Pharm.D., BC-ADM, FAPhA, FASHP, CDE
Educator/Clinician/Preceptor

*The mission of the playwright is to look in his heart and write, to write
whatever concerns him at the moment; to write with passion and conviction.
Of course the measure of the man will be the measure of the play.*

—Robert Anderson

Anderson's words strike a resonant chord within us as we reflect on what the practice of pharmacy means to us. Although
we are at very different stages of our careers, we share a similar
passion for our field and a deep responsibility for the people we
serve. John Boorman proposes, "What is passion? It is surely the
becoming of a person." We maintain that it is also the becoming of
a professional, a pharmacist, a clinician, and, ultimately a patient-
care advocate. Passion is needed in addition to our education and
training, because without it, we are mere dispensers of medication
and clinical medication management specialists.

John F. Kennedy said in a 1962 commencement address, "The
great enemy of the truth is very often not the lie—deliberate, contrived
and dishonest—but the myth—persistent, persuasive and unrealistic."
Some pharmacists believe the myth that we are limited in scope by how
others define the "role of a pharmacist," that we must always defer and
refer, that pharmacists are not "clinicians," or that our responsibility
ends with ensuring the right medication is given to the right patient.
Unfortunately, the two of us have each been held captive to this myth at
some point in our careers. By believing the myth, we pharmacists fail to
see the truth—that we can practice within interdisciplinary teams that

operate from a standpoint of mutual respect for the added value of each member's contributions to the team. The danger in failing to see the truth—in failing to act as patient care advocates—is that our patients pay the ultimate price. Each of us can provide evidence for that.

A Resident's Perspective: Dr. Yocum

For me, the initial cost was far too high. During my very first opportunity as a pharmacist to provide medical care for someone who would otherwise be without it, I did nothing. My failure occurred on my first APPE, a medical missions elective offered. Twenty-two students and three pharmacy faculty spent 10 days in Costa Rica running medical clinics assisted by three recent Costa Rican medical school graduates who served as translators. Three of those days were spent on Chira Island off the Pacific Coast—a 7-hour bus ride and a 2-hour boat ride. The remote location limited a physician to a 1-day annual visit to focus on treating the most acutely ill. Everyone lived in tents, but we were blessed to have running water and the minimum plumbing necessary to run the clinic. The mission group consisted of students ranging from P1s to P4s. Clerkship students helped lead the clinic and were each responsible for writing up a patient who was seen through the entire continuum of care—triage, medical examination, treatment recommendations, dispensing, counseling, and praying with each patient who welcomed it.

I assisted TP, a 30-year-old Hispanic woman with three children. She complained of severe abdominal pain that had been growing progressively worse for months. On the basis of a brief gynecological exam, the medical resident concluded that she had a vaginal infection that had likely progressed to pelvic inflammatory disease. He elected not to treat TP's infection because he wanted confirmation of the diagnosis, so he recommended to her that she follow up with a doctor on the mainland. Because I was afraid to speak up on her behalf, because I was unsure of my knowledge and skill set, because I believed I should defer to the medical resident's expertise, I said nothing. I said nothing, knowing that although we had medication to cover the spectrum of what was likely the cause of her infection, it did not consist of what would have been considered "first line" by the CDC. I said nothing, knowing that her husband was a fisherman who bartered with others on the island for the bare necessities for their family to survive. I said nothing, knowing that she would not be able to afford to go to the mainland for follow-up care. I dispensed ibuprofen for her pain and multivitamins for her and her children, prayed for her, and, 2 days later, left.

While developing my case presentation, the gnawing sensation in my stomach and the overwhelming guilt persisted; why hadn't I said anything? Couldn't we have given her something? Why hadn't I at least questioned the medical resident further about his reasons for referring her, about the consequences of not treating a known infection? I had traveled thousands of miles to help the less fortunate and found the measure of my role as pharmacist sorely lacking. When I gave my case presentation upon returning to the States, a professor was in attendance that had not accompanied us on the trip, but had experience with medical mission work as a leader. She asked me, "How do you feel about the fact that you may have been the only contact with a health care provider that woman will ever see, and you chose to do nothing?"

That question changed the course of my pharmacy career and my life. I found conviction and understood what it meant to have passion. Because of that question, I pursued this year of residency training. I hear that question in my mind every day and before every patient I see.

We have been blessed to continue our mission work domestically because of the indigent care clinical services established by Dr. Haines. As part of our residency program, residents are able to rotate through The Community Health Center (CHC) in West Palm Beach, Florida. It has afforded us the opportunity to continue to see patients for whom traditional health care is not an option, due in part to lack of citizenship or significant financial difficulties.

Our mission is to be patient care advocates while practicing pharmacy. Our measure is defined by the people, the patients we are able to see every day, *not* the number or manner of disease states.

A Preceptor's Perspective: Dr. Haines

Dr. Yocum insightfully demonstrates the need for passion in pharmacy practice. However, finding passion within ourselves solves only part of the equation. How do we inspire passion and conviction in the students we teach and precept? We can relay information, explain what it means to practice evidence-based medicine, and teach the critical thinking necessary to work through the many "gray areas" of practice. Yet how do we instill in students the ability to differentiate between seeing patients and being an advocate for patients? The answer put simply—we must create opportunities for them to experience it for themselves.

I recall my first patient, RC, in 2001, an elderly Jamaican woman who had not seen a physician in more than 10 years and therefore had not been appropriately screened for diabetes, hypertension, cholesterol, and heart disease based on her age, family history, and risk factors.

Our relationship blossomed, and through clinician coaching, RC's health greatly improved. The beauty of indigent care is that we are not constrained by traditional regulations, and I was able to spend as much time as necessary getting to know RC. I was able to treat her as a person and aid in the healing process that encompassed her emotional, spiritual, and physical health. Unfortunately, by the time she sought care with me, some damage could not be remedied, as her vision had suffered because of years of undiagnosed diabetes. As happens with so many patients here, I received the true blessing. Eventually, she was able to receive health care district aid and to transition from the clinic. Before leaving, she brought me a pink and blue crocheted potholder that was very intricate and detailed. This token of appreciation with her limited vision took almost a year for her to make. I keep the potholder in my office where I can see it daily as a constant symbolic reminder of our mission to serve others with our knowledge and expertise.

Conclusions

Our experiences have taught us that students' passion is ignited to the degree that preceptors allow them to manage patients as people first, disease states second. Unlike in other clinic settings, where there may be strict time constraints for appointments in place, an abundance of lab values useful for clinical monitoring, and a reliable method for referral or follow-up for patients, at CHC, our patients may be transient, and access to medications is challenging. Often, we will schedule a follow-up. Or in some cases, we finally receive the medication for them through patient assistance, and they never return. Which means that instead of just asking the students, "What would you recommend in an ideal setting," we are able to pose our own "classroom" assessment technique, the question that helped change Dr. Yocum's practice: "What will you do for this patient if you are the last health care provider they will see?" Will we initiate insulin without follow-up even though their hemoglobin A1C is 13.7%? Do we start the statin if we have no baseline LFTs or lipid panel? Will we initiate an ACEI or spironolactone without the ability to monitor potassium levels or renal function?

Several months ago in clinic, we saw a patient who presented with cellulitis. CJ had gone 2 years without any medication to treat his diabetes. It was one of those rare, unfortunate visits where we had to tell the patient that there was nothing we could do for him at our facility—he needed to go to the hospital immediately for treatment. When the two clerkship students present were asked the question, "What will you do for this patient," they replied with action, not words. They gave CJ the phone number to the clinic and instructed him to call that evening with his room number at the hospital (without being sure he would even follow our advice). The next day, the students called him at the hospital and spoke to CJ. They did this every day until he was discharged. When we were able to schedule follow-up care, we had to do so during our evening clinic because the students had already moved on to their next rotation; however, they had become so invested in CJ's care that they were willing to volunteer their time. Since our first encounter, CJ's diabetes is now controlled with the free insulin we are able to provide, and he has never missed an appointment. CJ lost his job and his home, but he found his spirit—and the students, their passion.

As we transition through our careers—as pharmacy student, resident, clinician, preceptor, researcher, academician, and perhaps more— we try to apply to our profession Anderson's words on the passion of the playwright: we look into our hearts and act on whatever concerns us at the moment; we act "with passion and conviction." We believe the measure of our careers and, by extension, ourselves, will be revealed in large part by how well we have practiced "with passion and conviction." As pharmacists, we will never waver in the degree of passion we express for our patients and foster in our students throughout our professional careers.

Deciphering the Code

Marianne E. Koenig, Pharm.D., BCPS
Academic and Research Fellow

It was unusually busy at the physician office that day, during my fourth week at this primary care rotation site. I so thoroughly enjoyed this rotation during my first year as an Academic and Research Fellow that I selected this site for my second-year elective rotation. Before this rotation, I had limited knowledge of, and experience with, the Medical Home Model of Primary Care. I was so impressed with the patient care outcomes produced by this practice site that I wanted to immerse myself and absorb any information I could to provide me ammunition to successfully practice in this setting after I completed my postdoctoral training. Because of my faculty mentor's confidence with my clinical and supervisory skills, she intentionally double-booked our patient appointments to maximize student–patient encounters. Days like these show students the skills of time management and keeping to the allotted appointment time, generating meaningful SOAP notes, and coordinating follow-up appointments with the staff, all while acting professionally. My faculty mentor was assisting a physician with a difficult medication before authorization, and I was charged with supervising the two professional year four (PY4) pharmacy students.

As our last patient consultation was concluding, one of the family practice physicians inquired if we could counsel one more patient. I immediately agreed, even though the students' heavy sighs and look of disappointment contradicted my enthusiasm. The physician picked up on their mannerisms and teased the two about being late for happy hour. The physician handed us the patient's chart, which indicated he was a 62-year-old African American male with diabetes. The PY4 students usually receive their assigned patient consultations a week prior to the scheduled appointment so that they can review the medical record and prepare a pharmacist care plan; however, this luxury of time was not possible. During the previous 3 weeks, my observations of their counseling of six diabetic patients gave me confidence that even without preparatory time, they would be capable of conducting a meaningful counseling session. I welcomed this unexpected referral, as it presented another opportunity for me to assess the students' critical thinking and communication skills.

The patient presented in disheveled, malodorous clothing. His hair was unkempt, and his face was unshaven. He wore long sleeves and slacks, even though it was topping 90 degrees outside. He walked slowly and deliberately as if he were favoring his left foot, similar to when you pull a calf muscle in one leg. I noticed his right shoe was untied and loosened. Our consultation room was very small, 4' × 6' at the most. I introduced myself and offered a handshake to our patient. I turned to the students and noted a hesitation to greet our patient, along with a lack of compassion in their voices and facial expressions. I sensed that their reluctance to greet our patient in the appropriate manner stemmed from the patient's appearance and odor.

The students proceeded with the consultation, asking straightforward, yes and no types of questions without depth like "Do you understand how your diabetes can affect other organs and nerves in your body?", "Have you ever had a hypoglycemic attack?", and "Have you missed any of your diabetes medication (pills or shots) within the past week?" Our patient disclosed that he had recently been released from a 30-year prison term, that he resided in public housing, and that he found it difficult to adhere to his oral and injectable diabetic regimen. Several times, I had to prompt the PY4 students to provide follow-up queries to statements made by our patient. For instance, the patient indicated he received most of his daily food intake from area soup kitchens. I asked both of the students, "Are you familiar with the typical food served at soup kitchens? How would you counsel our patient on controlling dietary factors if he is limited on food choices given his socioeconomic status?"

My impression was that the students were rushing the appointment, which was supported by the students not evaluating the patient's knowledge and perception of his disease and his rationale for his nonadherence. In addition, they failed to offer a foot examination. I was convinced this act was omitted on purpose for fear of the sight or smell they would encounter. After about 15 minutes, the patient indicated he had to leave because of his transportation issues. My gaze fell on the

PY4 students, and I was astonished to observe a look of joy. I attempted to compose myself while politely recommending to the patient that we schedule a comprehensive follow-up appointment to coincide with his hemoglobin A1C results, which were due back in a few days. He agreed to return in 1 week to meet with both of the PY4 students and me.

While I escorted our patient to the waiting room, I clearly over-heard one of the students say, "Thank goodness that is over. I was so nervous he was going to ask for my wallet." The other student respond-ed no better with, "I'll find out when his next appointment is so we can plan on calling in sick." Debriefing with the students occurs after each patient encounter. I felt that I had to refrain from saying how I really felt about their behavior during the consultation: that it was judgmental, callous, cold, and pretentious. I literally had to leave the room to gather my thoughts. I am certain their pharmacy curriculum provided ample opportunity to learn and apply the principles of the "Code of Ethics for Pharmacists" and "Oath of a Pharmacist" to patient-centered care. My disappointment with their conduct almost brought me to tears. Is it the "millennial" factor? How could these "20-somethings" have completed more than 6 years of higher education and still stereotype? More impor-tantly, how could I convince these pharmacy students of their profes-sional obligation to treat all patients equally with respect and dignity? Once my pulse slowed down, I entered the room, paused, and decided to take a completely different trajectory with my debriefing session.

I asked the students to recite the Pharmacist Code of Ethics & Oath. Their looks of puzzlement and their silence were disheartening. After roughly 60 seconds without any response, I informed the PY4s that to-morrow, we would have a working lunch break, during which we would discuss their personal reflections of this patient encounter. I instructed them to prepare a two-page reflection telling of their encounter with this patient and supporting or contradicting the themes of the Pharma-cist Code of Ethics & Oath.

I was distraught. I am not sure which upset me more—their behavior during the encounter or their lack of recognizing the key principles from the Oath and Code. I wanted to scream. I gathered my belongings and fled the office without even acknowledging the students or my faculty mentor. Campus was 7 blocks away. The solitude during my brisk walk allowed some self-reflection. With fresh air in my lungs, I sensed clarity to the basis of my emotions. My actions directed toward the students mimicked the student–patient interaction I had just witnessed. I was so focused on proving that their behaviors were a product of their generation instead of evaluating their comprehension of the behaviors expected of health care professionals. My attitudes toward the students influenced my behavior. I felt defeated. I had failed as an instructor. Why did I neglect to provide the necessary feedback, which these two students desperately needed? That evening, I obsessed about my actions during and after the patient encounter. Should I have halted the consultation and brought the two students into the hall to redirect their actions? Why did I not address their inappropriate behaviors immediately after the appointment? What kind of example was I portraying by fleeing from a difficult issue? Why did I not seek advice from my faculty mentor?

After an unsuccessful night of sleep, I arose early with a sense of urgency to construct my own reflection of the disappointment I experienced with my lack of instruction. I recognized that my emotions precluded me from objectively assessing the students' performance. How can I improve on this trait? I realized that by delaying my feedback to the two PY4s, I was able to prevent a potential unprofessional debrief. In fact, I recalled that last year, during my first year of the Fellowship, I received criticism from one faculty preceptor in a very condescending manner. I had written and submitted to my faculty preceptor for review what I thought was a very thorough SOAP note. I was shocked to have my SOAP note critiqued in a very negative manner in the presence of PY4 students. As a practicing pharmacist for 17 years before pursuing my postdoctoral training, I value feedback for improving my communication skills; however, I would have appreciated the opportunity to discuss my writing in private and not to have been subjected to a mini-lecture on "everything wrong with the SOAP note." I strive to provide a nurturing, positive learning environment, not to teach with the negativity I witnessed as a Fellow. In retrospect, I am grateful for delaying the students' debriefing, which thus allowed me to prepare for objective and constructive advice delivered in a professional manner. Finally, I realized that their inexperience was the root cause of my emotional state. I am 20 years their senior and need to remember they are still learning. The students need continual guidance and opportunities to practice the principles from the Oath and Code.

That afternoon, I began the debriefing session by explaining my reason for the delay. I acknowledged that I was overcome with emotion from my observation of their verbal and nonverbal behaviors. In addition, I stated that I had overheard their comments at the end of the consultation, specifically about stereotyping our patient. I explained to them how I felt their behaviors contradicted key principles from the Oath and Code. I illustrated my point by indicating where I felt they were deficient. Respecting a patient's autonomy and dignity, along with showing moral and ethical conduct, was absent during their patient encounter. I admitted to the students that my emotional reaction from their behavior affected my judgment in providing a clear identification of the learning outcomes and the rationale for the reflection assignment. I shared with them my journey of self-reflection from my personal experiences with negative feedback to the realization that PY4 students have not experienced enough real-world opportunities to apply the principles of the Oath and Code. Furthermore, I indicated that I should have communicated my concerns before they departed from the physician office. They admitted to me that they had never before interacted with a patient with poor hygiene or with an ex-convict.

Although their personal reflections assignment did not successfully address their lack of ethical and professional behaviors, they both verbally acknowledged understanding that their actions during the previous day's encounter did not uphold key principles of being a professional pharmacist. They indicated they were embarrassed that I overheard their comments about "calling in sick" and "stealing their wallet" and that they never meant for the patient to be treated any differently because of his socioeconomic situation. After dissecting each of the questions asked during the encounter and identifying more appropriate questioning techniques, we concluded the debriefing session. I felt satisfied that they recognized areas in need of improvement. Also, I felt satisfied enough about the process of my own continuous quality improvement that I could recognize opportunities to enhance my teaching and communication skills. From this encounter with that elderly gentleman with diabetes, I have grown a little, both personally and professionally.

Humbled by Haiti

Shari Allen, Pharm.D.
PGY 2 Psychiatric Pharmacy Resident

S aying I like to give back or do community service is an under-statement. When I was a child, I was the first person in the class to volunteer to help the teacher with activities. When I turned 16 and started driving, I kept bags of food in my car for homeless people. When I went to college, I spent a good amount of my free time volunteering in soup kitchens, and when I was in pharmacy school, I helped start a scholarship foundation for the classes that were graduating after me. Volunteering or giving back is my personal high. It makes me feel good. I get a rush out of doing things for others. Sure, I believe giving back is the right thing to do, but I have to admit, volunteering used to be more about me and what I got out of it. All of this changed on August 7, 2010, when I left for my first day of a medical mission trip to Port-au-Prince, Haiti.

After the earthquake in Haiti, I knew there would be an opportunity to volunteer. I prayed on ways that I could help or be of assistance. I gave money through various foundations. This still was not enough to give me long-term gratification. Then, somewhat randomly, I received an e-mail from Project Medishare, which was looking for pharmacists to come help at a hospital in Port-au-Prince, a perfect opportunity for me. I had to take a week off from my residency, which I cleared with my residency director, and against the will of some of my family and friends, I was on a plane headed to Haiti.

I did not know exactly what I was going to be doing there as a pharmacist, so I came up with my own ideas. I thought, how great will this be? I'm going to help save lives, rebuild buildings, and help feed or clothe people in need. I thought, I am going to go there and save the day (all of this gives me the rush that I like to feel when volunteering). Looking back at it, I'm actually ashamed that I made this opportunity more about me and less about the people I was there to help—and little did I know that I was going to be the one on the receiving end of that help.

When I landed in Port-au-Prince, I was escorted to the hospital site. Along with the other volunteers (of various medical professions), I was immediately given my assignment. I would be staffing in the pharmacy for the week. This meant I was not going to have quite the impact I thought I would. I headed to the pharmacy to see my schedule and was surprised to learn that I would be working an overnight shift (7:00 p.m.–7:00 a.m.) on my first day. The pharmacy was about the size of my bedroom back at home, 13 × 16. It lacked some of the accommodations I was used to, but oddly, I felt comfortable. The walls were the same drab off-white of my office in the States, but unlike my office, it had a large window that allowed me to see the people on the streets of Haiti and the sunlight, which was my indicator that the shift would soon be over. All of us volunteers were warned about the continuous rain, the heat, and the gnats; they didn't mention the mice (which we named Bob) and lizards (Joe) that frequented the walls and floors of the pharmacy. Despite our friends, Bob and Joe, the pharmacy became the place to be in the hospital; we were the only unit with a working air conditioner (when the power wasn't out) and a water cooler. There were four large shelves of various medications, all donated. The pharmacist in charge was a compounding pharmacist in the States, so we had a decent supply of compounding tools. The refrigerator was stocked with Ativan vials, propofol, and other IV medications. My biggest responsibilities were going to be to supply the emergency room with the medications they needed overnight and to prepare and deliver the IV medications needed most frequently by the pediatric unit. Throughout the week, I would be working alongside one of the Haitian pharmacists and a local technician. Being the person who loves to save the day, I thought this would be a great opportunity to show each of them what I learned in pharmacy school and how I could possibly help them run their pharmacy better. I walked into my shift that night thinking, I'm in charge here.

The hospital was the only one in Port-au-Prince with a fully functioning emergency room. Patients would be brought from all over Haiti. Armed guards at the gate acted as the triage; they would determine who could be treated and who would need to wait. It seemed like everyone decided to have an emergency the night I was working. Within the same hour, we admitted a woman with severe labor pains, a man with congestive heart failure, a construction worker who fell off the top floor of a building, and several premature babies with seizures and respiratory failure. Orders began to come in from the ER at a quick pace.

They were calling for multiple morphine drips and various IV antibiotics (all of which needed to be reconstituted), and they were asking for recommendations based on what they wanted to give the patient and what we had available in the pharmacy. Many of the pediatric patients needed IV antiseizure medications STAT, which also needed to be calculated for a pediatric dose. While this was going on, the nurses from the other units at the hospital were coming in and taking the oral medications they needed for their patients. Everything was happening all at once, and I began to panic. I remembered why I suffered through my ER rotation; people needed answers, medications—things now, not tomorrow. For the first time as a pharmacist, I felt like I could really hurt someone if I didn't get this right. This added pressure caused my anxiety to kick in. My breath became labored, my heart was racing, my mind was foggy, and the tears were starting to flow. I was doubting my abilities as a pharmacist. I kept thinking, I'm struggling with things that should be second nature to me by now (i.e., metric conversions). Trissel's and Micromedex became my best friends during this trip. Unfortunately, the ER and pediatric patients could not wait for me to look up information. I had to rely on the Haitian staff more than I initially wanted to. After all, wasn't I supposed to be the one saving the day?

After my first shift ended, I went back to my room and thought about what I could teach everyone to do during the next shift so that things would run smoother. Then I realized, it's not they who need the help, it's me. I needed to be real with myself. I had to be able to admit that I don't know everything and that it's okay to ask for help. As someone who likes to be the person to fix things and be in control (all of the time), I find that asking for help can be hard to do. I remember e-mailing my mother, telling her how I lost complete control of the pharmacy because I was trying to be the hero. I wasn't in Haiti to be a hero; I was there to help in whatever way they saw fit. In my case, it was staffing the pharmacy. After all the volunteers leave, the Haitian pharmacists, nurses, doctors, occupational therapist, etc., were going to be running the hospital themselves.

As medical professionals volunteering in a foreign environment, we have to realize that we need to be assisting them in operating their hospital, and if there are any ideas that come up in the process, then we can share and teach. If we go to their facility and try to take over and be the hero, in the long run, everyone loses. I was supposed to be teaching the Haitian technician some of the skills needed as a pharmacist. She genuinely wanted to learn; unfortunately, I let that night in the pharmacy get the best of me, and we both walked away with a bad experience.

This trip, however, was amazing. It taught me so many things. After I let go of my need to be the one helping everyone, the rest of the trip went by much smoother. Over the next week, I learned how to do IV compounding in an easier way. I learned how to rely less on the apps on my iPod and more on the information I learned while in pharmacy school. I learned about so many drugs that I'm not exposed to on a normal basis at my hospital in the States. Most importantly, because of this experience (along with the struggles), I have now challenged myself never to stop learning, to see every situation as a learning opportunity (not just in a classroom setting), and to be a better pharmacist.

Although my intentions were good when I went to Haiti, I was initially going for me and for what I could do for them. When I was able (or forced) to let that go, it became an experience that allowed me to take away much more than I thought I would. Had I not let go of my ego, I would have never been open to learning half of the things that I did. People always ask me if I would go back. The answer is yes. Although I still believe I have so much to give as a volunteer, I now know that I have even more to gain.

Educational Care

Teaching, Mentoring, and Learning

To me the sole hope of human salvation lies in teaching.

George Bernard Shaw

Good teaching cannot be reduced to technique; good teaching comes from the identity and integrity of the teacher.

Parker J. Palmer

Life is a learning experience, only if you learn.

Yogi Berra

Stay Cool: Springtime in Academia

Kimberly A. Pesaturo, Pharm.D., BCPS
Educator

It was still wintertime, but we were calling it "early" spring semester. Notoriously my busiest semester, the impending spring always brought mild feelings of panic, knowing that I was entering into a 4-month commitment of 70- to 80-hour workweeks, various courses to teach, and seemingly, minimal time spent with my husband and young, formative child. This particular spring was the most emotionally draining in my memory because it started with an experience with a student named Elise.

To spare the situational details and maintain my pact of confidentiality with Elise, the vague version of this story will have to suffice. In short, neither of us had a particularly easy time on her APPE (advanced pharmacy practice experience) clinical rotation. Elise was a challenge for me as an educator and in my clinical practice environment; a busy critical care–focused site was a challenge for her as well. I attributed her non-motivation to lack of interest, or lack of caring, or lack of sleep, depending on the day or her excuse. Naïvely, I never attributed her anti-work attitude toward me, because this was the first time an experience like this had happened in several years and countless clinical rotations with students.

The snow was terrible this particular winter and led to several missed rotation days. On other days, I had to drive in with a friend who had all-wheel drive just to make it to work safely. We were anxiously waiting for spring, or more accurately, we would have all been okay if spring had just quickly moved into next semester's summer.

Over 6 weeks of clinical education, the situation with Elise grew increasingly more difficult for both of us. Her third-week rotation evaluation reflected a mash-up of the time we had together between snow cancellations. Her next weekly rotation evaluation became a prolonged event that evolved from the passing down of a poor mid-point grade, to tears and repentance, to a plan to move forward in a transforming manner. We would conquer this together; we would overcome Elise's non-attempts to work, because in the end, I was an educator with a perceived commitment to success and could "break through" to anyone if I tried really hard. Elise agreed; she wanted success and she wanted motivation. We started to see the warmer weather together for the first time.

Optimistically, we decided to move forward into the last few weeks of the semester. The next day, Elise arrived to rotation dressed in a professional white coat, but also in sneakers and jeans. Later, she pulled me aside one day to ask the interpretation of patient data. I asked her to look it up and report back. She never did. Elise continued to arrive late to our clinical meetings. We said we would meet at 9:00 a.m. At 9:25 a.m. on a particular Thursday, a colleague of mine saw Elise walk into our unit. Frustrated by her late arrival, he immediately yelled, "Get out." On the second-to-last day of the rotation, she presented a case that she had fabricated. Final evaluations would be reviewed the following day, and I told Elise that I could not allow her to pass the rotation. I had not given her a formal grade at that point, but in hindsight, I think my preemptive warning was more out of frustration than concern. Elise asked me to reconsider, telling me that I could allow her to pass if I wanted. I had to shake my head and say, "But, I can't." Many words unspoken, Elise simply walked out that afternoon in silent tears.

It snowed again the night before final evaluations, and I prayed that school would be cancelled. I did not want to face what I had to do with this student. At 10:00 that night, I was as awake as if I had just had a large coffee, so I called a trusted colleague at home, knowing he would be up. He talked to me for over an hour.

"You are doing the right thing," he said.

"It would be a disservice to the profession and to the student to inflate the grade so she passes," he said.

"It is part of our professional obligation to educate and assess; you've done that, and now all you are doing is applying the appropriate consequences," he said.

I thanked him profusely and hung up the phone sometime between 11 p.m. and midnight.

I think I fell asleep somewhere around 2:00 a.m. At 3:00 a.m., my young daughter woke up and wanted to sleep in my bed. She did not fall back to sleep until 5:00 a.m. At 6:00 a.m., my alarm went off, and I got ready for the day.

I could not muster the energy to fix my hair or apply my makeup. After all, I was about to go and break the news to a student that we had failed, but she would be the one suffering the consequences. I drove to work in a daze, consumed by thoughts of the following: the reaction of her parents when she broke the news that she would not graduate on time; the impact on her career that deferring a job acceptance might bring; the fact that she would probably destroy me on my own evaluation, thus tarnishing what I had worked so hard to protect.

At 8:00 a.m., I walked into my office building and was met by a senior colleague, who had agreed to sit in on this student's final evaluation with me.

"You are doing the right thing," she said. "If you have been up front with this student about her performance throughout the rotation, this should come as no surprise to her. I'm sure you have the documentation to support everything you've told me."

As the student walked in, I was in a panic. Documentation? I did have that, right? Had I told the student enough? Did she know?

"Elise, thank you for joining us today. Unfortunately, we have to tell you that the outcome of the rotation is failure."

Elise replied slowly, her eyes puffy from either crying or sleeplessness, "I...had...no...idea..."

We discussed her lateness; she did not think it was a big deal. We discussed her unprofessionalism; she said she was never taught that she was unprofessional on any previous rotation. She asked why I did not tell her any of this earlier; she had focused on my optimism that we could fix this together. But, I had told her. Why hadn't she listened?

Pages of data and my own notes spoke for themselves. This was not something I was *doing* to the student, I repeatedly explained. This was simply my objective reaction to the student's performance. The conversation circled for a while. Eventually, Elise politely excused herself and left, silent and head down as she walked out of my office.

I left early that morning, too. I walked back to my car through the dirty, slushy snow. I needed sleep and had no further appointments that day. I was sure I had just ruined Elise's life, so I could think of nothing else to do that day but to ruminate over my own failure as a teacher.

Time eventually healed my perception of the situation, and subsequent groups of rotation students fared significantly better. In hindsight, out of countless "A" grades handed out to students, I had never previously learned the true meaning of documentation and fair and unbiased assessment. However, Elise's situation prompted some questions: would better assessment have prevented her failure? Or, did Elise receive the grade she had earned, and my pages of documentation were simply, and luckily, the result of my naïve note-taking? With one failure (my own or Elise's, I was never sure), I was taught the value of assessment. Formative assessment, snapshot pieces to constantly assess student learning, became the focus of my process. I altered the manner in which I provided feedback; we went from the old weekly system to the daily feedback approach. Rubrics became a way of life on my rotation. Not only would I provide constant and unbiased feedback to the students, but I would ask them to assess each other as well. As I met with students for their formal grade feedback, I asked them first to tell me what grade they thought they had earned, and to justify why this was the case. Most of them guessed low, out of humility, I suppose.

My documentation quickly became flawless and my agenda, transparent. Grades were, I assured the students, never a reaction to an emotional process. They were simply a reflection of the student's performance, based on an up-front set of criteria. I simply served to facilitate this process and hopefully teach something along the way.

On a particularly warm day months later, I received a note from Elise. Elise was completing her makeup summer rotation, weeks after her colleagues had graduated. The note was brief, but it stated the following: "Dear Dr. P— Thank you for teaching me a true lesson. Stay cool." I laughed at the irony here and simply responded, "And to you, the same."

The Perfect Patient

Adrienne J. Lindblad, Pharm.D., BSP, BSc, ACPR
Clinician/Preceptor

Sometimes, the answers to our problems are staring us in the face. Like many preceptors, I have continually been baffled by how much "work" it is to precept students. They take up so much time and energy, and I am exhausted by the time their rotation is complete. After all, it takes a lot of effort to plan rotation activities, create a schedule, orient the students to my practice, and then actively supervise the students, assign their patient load, and answer their questions.

When I take students, I know I am contributing to the education of the next generation of pharmacists. I know that precepting is a great way to recruit future staff. I know that students allow me to reflect on ways to improve my own practice and provide me with the opportunity to learn from them. But sometimes, the workload is so demanding that I am not always sure the experience of "precepting" is as rewarding as I am told it is.

On any given day, I have 36 patients on my hospital unit to care for, and I can barely provide the level of care that I want to for a mere fraction of these patients. When I have students, suddenly I am expected to integrate them to my practice area, get to know them and their preferred learning style, provide feedback, and review all the work the student does for that patient. It is exhausting, and I wonder if it interferes with my ability to care for my patients. I want students to help me in my practice, not hinder me.

It's not that I don't try to be a good preceptor. I want the students' experience to be positive. I want students to learn everything they can while they are with me, and I want them to enjoy their rotation so much that they choose a career in hospital practice. As a result, I try to review my list of new admissions in the morning and quickly review their medications before assigning patients to students to ensure that the student cares for patients with the "right" level of complexity. We don't want to give a student a patient who is severely demented or aggressive or one who has too many comorbidities, for example.

So, you can imagine how I was feeling one morning when I was just way too busy to take the time to find the "right" patient for my final-year practicum student who was just starting her hospital rotation. I just randomly picked a patient and told her to "just go with it." I already expect my students to independently develop a workup of their patients and then provide me with a verbal, structured summary of the patient and their pharmacy care plan. A few hours later, the student came to me with a very thick patient chart and a stack of her own notes, looking like a deer in the headlights. "I don't know where to start" was all she could say. It turned out the patient I assigned had a very long admission history, including numerous emergency surgeries with many complications and a tracheostomy; the patient was also newly nonverbal and depressed, with multiple comorbidities. I felt awful. I thought this was very complex, even for an experienced hospital pharmacist. It was definitely not fair for a student to be responsible for this patient!

However, I did not have the time to find a more suitable patient for the student. Additionally, this patient was clearly experiencing drug-related issues that I did not have the time to resolve. So, instead, I spent about 10 minutes explaining to the student how I would approach this case: where I would start, how I would gather her entire complex history, how I would break up the current issues the patient was experiencing into manageable "chunks," and how I would prioritize the issues based on severity and patient wishes. I explained that the basic approach to providing a workup for a patient is always the same, but sometimes, it just takes longer to do.

The student still had some trepidation, but she went away to complete her workup. A few hours later, she was presenting all of her patients to me. When we got to this patient, she presented the patient and a well-thought-out preliminary care plan for the patient. She had a lot of learning to do about the patient's various conditions, but she prioritized what to learn first based on the severity of the issue. I was shocked. No, I was impressed. Here was this extremely complex patient, and my student had a plan to care for this patient. Why had I been wasting my time worrying about finding the perfect patient? The perfect patient for a student is a patient the student can learn from. That means any patient is the perfect patient.

I have since applied this concept of "any patient" to at least six other students. To date, all of them have been successful. There haven't been any tears, and there's been no whining about workload or the complexity of the patients. In fact, my students have commented on how they appreciate the opportunity to care for "real" patients; patients with complex issues and sometimes strange and rare conditions; patients that the students will be responsible for once they graduate from pharmacy school in a few short months.

So, here I had this problem of feeling students were a hindrance to me in my practice. Now, with this small change in my attitude, students are a welcome relief. Together, we provide care for more patients, and I am not feeling as overwhelmed. Students actually help me out. Do other student health professionals pick and choose which patients they care for? No, they care for any and all patients, and that is what student pharmacists should do. It is our duty to provide care for whoever needs it. The people who are most at risk of experiencing drug-related issues and who are in greatest need of our help are often the most sick and complex patients we see. These patients provide a wealth of learning opportunities for our students and allow students to see the true nature of patient care in a hospital setting. Students are ready for the challenge. The sooner we can trust our students' skills and abilities, the sooner they will be an asset to our practice.

Put the Magic in the Beginning

Roger W. Sommi, Pharm.D., FCCP, BCPP
Educator

When I was in fellowship training in the mid-1980s, one of the opportunities afforded me was to work with doctor of pharmacy students on clerkship. Back then, these students were postbaccalaureate, motivated, and bright—the best of the best. The majority of Pharm.D. programs at that time were 2-year postbaccalaureate programs. Commonly, these programs were structured as 1 year of intensive didactic instruction followed by 12 months of clerkship. There was one Pharm.D. student who dramatically changed the way I approach teaching students. She simply said to me after rounds one day, "How did you do that?" "How did you figure out what the problem was with that patient?" I was taken aback by the question. Surely everyone knew how to do it, I thought to myself. She went on to explain that she had been on clerkship for many months and could answer any question that came up on rounds, but she did not feel like she understood how the whole thing worked; the ability to assess patients and come up with recommendations was still mysterious and magical to her. She had been following around some of the most notable pharmacy practitioners on previous clerkships, and she was amazed at how they could identify these important drug problems in patients. She wanted me to show her the secret.

I went on to draw out a huge diagram on the chalkboard of one patient—essentially delineating all the information I thought was important about that patient, the connections between the data and the patient, and the advantages and disadvantages of each of the choices we had at every step of the process. Together, we listed what information we knew about the patient—diagnosis, labs, medications, progress to date, and remaining issues to resolve. We decided we really didn't need more information at this point to move forward. We identified what we wanted to accomplish by making a change in drug therapy and identified all the potential options—from the traditional forms of intervention to wild combinations—all of which came from our collective knowledge of the literature. We began a detailed discussion of pros and cons for each potential intervention and settled on one—the one I had earlier recommended on rounds. It struck me that what I had just written on the board was the process by which I took care of patients' problems, but it was something that I did automatically, not being fully aware of every detail along the way. The only thing this student wanted me to do was simply to think out loud.

A few years later, Strand and colleagues[1] published a paper describing the structure and function of drug-related problems. They described eight categories of drug-related problems—and argued that the scope of pharmacists' practice revolved around finding and solving these problems. This was the last piece of the puzzle for me in teaching students. Students simply needed to understand that what we do as pharmacists is find and solve these drug-related problems.

I teach an hour-long discussion on drug-related problems in the introductory course during the first semester of the first year for pharmacy students. We review the descriptions of each different type of problem and come up with examples of each type and the ways it might affect patient outcome. At the end of the lecture, I advise them that they should look at each of the courses that follow in the curriculum through the lens of these problems. I also make a promise—that any student who sees me on clerkship will be asked—"What do pharmacists do?" and "What are the eight drug-related problems?" So far, I have kept that promise.

Fast forward to introductory clerkship. Students show up on their first day, hopeful to see patients and make a difference in the world. I know I have to show them some of the magic of what we do as practitioners. I tell them that the first thing I want them to do is review the chart of a patient who has come and gone—to get a perspective on what we do at the hospital. At the end of the review, I simply want them to tell me about their patient in a 5-minute or less presentation to me on a pharmacist-to-pharmacist level. I ask them to make believe they are going off service, I am coming on service, and they need to tell me what I need to know about the patient to continue their care.

Like clockwork, they diligently read every word in the chart in preparation to tell me exactly what happened. Being in psychiatry is helpful here because the stories are often very colorful. Generally, I give them as long as they want—and they usually take 1.5–2 hours. They each dutifully present their patients, easily completing within the 5-minute limit. Without fail, over several years of this exercise, these students present much of the detail of the circumstances of the patient's admission. We hear about the police bringing the patient to the emergency room, or the unusual behaviors the patient displayed, and descriptions of hallucinations and delusional thinking. I prod them, hoping to hear the information I need to begin making decisions about these patients. But alas, I don't get it. Few or none of the data that practitioners need to make decisions about drug therapy are presented—you know—allergies, hepatic function, renal function, age, weight, diagnosis...and sometimes, they even forget drug doses and regimens! I have stopped being disappointed—this happens every year—and I now look at it as an opportunity to teach the students something about who they are as pharmacists and what responsibility they have for the patient.

I ask them—What do pharmacists do? They look sheepishly at each other—and eventually one of them comes up with the right answer—we find and solve drug-related problems. We go on to list each one. And I ask them—Do you have the right information to answer questions about each of these? How do you know they are actually receiving the right drug? Do you know if they are not allergic to the drug (wrong drug)? Are there interactions? Are they on too high a dose or too low a dose? Did you look for evidence of adverse reactions? Do they have a medical condition for which they are not receiving drug therapy? HOW DO YOU KNOW?

I ask each of them to begin to identify the "need to know" and "nice to know" information pharmacists need to begin our work. We list each of the suggestions on the board and, as a group, decide whether we need to know this or whether it is just nice to know. They can easily identify what information is needed and begin to prioritize the data based on the need to know/nice to know dichotomy. It is personally rewarding to see the light bulbs light up when they begin to see the path of the process. I think it is critical to the students' learning for them to do first what comes naturally to them in order for them to understand where they are in grasping the skills associated with the process of taking care of patients. Simply giving them a form to fill out keeps them in the dark about why they are doing it.

It occurs to me that we as teachers do not spend much, if any, time with students teaching *all* the processes involved in managing patients' medication therapy. Certainly, we provide extensive levels of knowledge and even challenge them with multiple cases and case discussions. What we fail to do is tell them how we constructed the case and gathered the information. We present the case; describe what additional details might be needed to better delineate the drug problems; and discuss the goals of treatment, selection of treatment, and monitoring of outcome. But where is it that we teach students how to gather information and organize it in a meaningful way? Clearly, this should be part of the initial part of teaching them the process of finding and solving drug-related problems—well before they begin working cases in pharmacotherapy or seeing patients on clerkship.

1. Strand LM, Morley PC, Cipolle R, Ramsey R, Lamsam GD. Drug-related problems: Their structure and function. DICP 1990;24:1093–7.

The Value of Information: A Wake-Up Call

Alex Flannery, Pharm.D.
Student

At some point, I imagine we all encounter a patient we will never forget. Someone who changes the way we view ourselves as health care professionals and, more importantly, changes the way we practice.

My wake-up call came halfway through my final year of rotations and on my second week of an internal medicine experience at an academic medical center. Our team was rounding on a middle-aged cirrhotic man who was awaiting placement to a rehabilitation center secondary to a fall from his hospital bed. For the week that I had known the patient, he was usually lying back in his hospital bed, and he gave us a smile when the team entered the room. Now, something was different. The patient was sitting straight up. His tense face had an angry expression etched onto it, and tears were visible out of the corners of his eyes.

"This is horrible. I'm just so frustrated. I was just talking to my family and couldn't explain anything. They're asking me when I'm leaving the hospital and about all of these medicines I'm taking and I have no idea what anything is for."

He didn't understand why he was taking lactulose or how it worked. He was bewildered about why he was taking propranolol, a blood pressure medication, when he did not have hypertension. He did not understand why a nurse was giving him subcutaneous injections in his abdomen, nor could he recall his antibiotic or its dosage. The inability to communicate his medication regimen to his family had brought him to tears.

Enter the pharmacy student. From my days of community practice to this very day, I still have never seen a patient so grateful for something so simple: information. I spoke with the medical team regarding the patient's discharge plan and made a list of all of his current medications and those he would likely be taking at the rehabilitation center. The list included indication, potential adverse effects, and expected duration of therapy. Then I discussed with the patient the importance of titrating lactulose to bowel movements, something he was unaware of. He had never been told that lactulose was for preventing his portal systemic encephalopathy, or even that the medication was going to cause him to have more frequent bowel movements. We reviewed other indications for his therapy, including propranolol for his variceal hemorrhage prophylaxis, spironolactone for his fluid retention, and the course of levofloxacin he was finishing for a urinary tract infection. I explained why it was so important that nurses provide him his subcutaneous injections of enoxaparin, with his recent fracture and reduced mobility.

I had wrongly assumed that a patient with a chronic disease would understand his medication therapy. I also assumed other bedside health care professionals would answer the patient's medication-related questions as drugs were being administered. My total interaction with this patient took only 30 minutes, during which we were able to review all of his medications and address all of his concerns. A smile and a handshake later, I could see the frustrations fading away, and he kept his medication list on his tray table for the remainder of his hospital stay. Whether or not my interaction with him gave him a sense of control, I will never know. One thing I do know is that I will never forget him.

I was used to rounding on patients, making daily medication changes, and providing discharge counseling. My experience with this man served as a not-so-gentle wake-up call of what it must be like to have your medications changed daily with little explanation. I assumed that the patient knew what his cirrhosis medications were for and, beyond this, that an in-house patient awaiting transfer would likely be the last person to have medication-related questions. I sensed the patient's frustration and saw a lack of knowledge quickly spiral into a perceived lack of control.

I had always been taught to empower patients. My pharmacy school lectures always stressed the importance of empowering outpatients and improving outcomes. When I was in community practice, I observed pharmacists empowering patients constantly by giving them choices about their medications as well as educating them regarding indications, expected duration of therapy, and potential adverse effects. This patient caused me to stop and think: Was I empowering my patients during their hospital stay? Or was I helping to depersonalize inpatient medicine? Was I treating the patient like a puzzle, an inanimate object from which I took away and added pieces to achieve an end point? As the saying goes, "Knowledge is power. Information is power."

This patient changed my view of inpatient pharmacy practice. Before this experience, I believed the optimal time for an inpatient clinical pharmacist to interact with patients was on admission and before discharge. I now believe this is the minimum that I should strive for. Now, if the team makes significant medication changes to the patient's regimen, I will stop in a patient's room, reintroduce myself as the pharmacy student on the team, review some of the patient's recent medication changes, and ask if they have any questions. I was not entirely sure what to expect when I started doing this, but I have no regrets. More often than not, whether it be a therapy change never discussed with them, questions about what different intravenous medications are for, or requests that a home medication be restarted, patients will have something that I can help them with. I am able to get to know my patients better and, at the same time, feel like I am contributing to their care.

This experience taught me that I want to empower patients to take an active role in discussing daily medication changes. Implementing a practice setting where the pharmacist is a constant source of drug information for the patient has the potential to change the perception of inpatient pharmacy, and more importantly, it can empower patients during a hospital stay by increasing their awareness of their medication regimen. In doing so, my hope is that I can help prepare patients for discharge sooner. If they feel in control of their medications, it is one less barrier to stop them from going home. "Knowledge is power. Information is power."

Growing Confidence STAT: Mentorship in the Emergency Room

Kelly Kabat, Pharm.D., BCPS
Student

What influences the success of a person? There are many factors, including personal drive, work ethic, and a quality support system. As I have learned, mentors are one of the most important influences on helping young pharmacy professionals grow into excellent pharmacists.

I was blessed as a student to rotate through areas with some of the most energetic, smart, and fun pharmacists I have ever worked with. For one of my final student rotations, I managed to wiggle my way into an emergency department rotation as the first student of a young pharmacist, Brett, who was still building this new area of practice. From the first day, the relationships he had built with the physicians, residents, and nurses in less than a year were evident. They trusted him and came to him frequently with questions or concerns. In the same way, he put his trust in me to learn as much as I could and work on building similar relationships.

Within the first half hour of arriving on my first day, we were already in a room preparing to intubate a patient with severe respiratory disease. He said, "Draw up 1.5 mg/kg of succinylcholine and 2 mg/kg of ketamine." I almost froze trying to calculate the dose and divide it by the concentration on the bottles as I stared at the syringe and needle, not even knowing what these drugs were. Somehow, I managed to say the dose of each while he drew it up and handed it to the physicians. In contrast to my panic, his calmness and efficiency were important for me to see. The multitude of lessons learned in those first few minutes I still carry with me today. I never forgot those drugs or the dosages, and more importantly, I know the value of taking a deep breath and having confidence in yourself to do what needs to be done for the patient in stressful situations.

A couple of weeks later, a young woman not much older than I am came into the emergency department with difficulty breathing due to terminal metastatic lung cancer. She was married with two young children and was hoping to stay alive long enough for her extended family to say their goodbyes. One of the ED physicians was going to place a chest tube and wanted the pharmacist to help with the conscious sedation. My job was to observe the procedure from the sidelines. As we were entering the room, the physician carried a chair and set it in the corner for me in case I needed to sit down while watching. After the procedure started, it was clear that this was going to be slightly more complicated than the usual chest tube because of the massive amounts of scar tissue surrounding her lungs. The nurse was working hard, trying to tend to the patient directly as well as making sure the doctor was getting everything she needed. Brett was trying to keep the patient as comfortable as possible with the medications, but as you can imagine, the prolonged procedure was painful; she would occasionally try to reach toward the pain, and he would gently hold her hand down. Quickly, I was no longer a student standing on the edge, but a member of the team trying to help this patient. My job was to hold the patient's hand and help pull instruments from drawers for the doctor. Brett drew up medications and helped the nurse with suctioning the patient. Eventually, the tube was stitched into place, and the patient was admitted to the hospital.

By not only watching, but also playing a small part in the care of this patient, I participated in the same routine that I was noticing over and over in the care of patients who came into the emergency department. One major part of the routine was teamwork. Everyone worked together, and the line of "whose job was whose" often blended, especially between the nurses and pharmacists. For example, we would often prepare medications such as antibiotics for the nurses as they were ordered by the physician, but Brett would often go beyond this and prepare the pumps and tubing if the nurse was busy so that the medication could get started right away.

My preceptor continued to push me during those 4 weeks in the emergency department, requiring the best of me at all times. I had daily readings every night about emergency medicine topics with indepth discussions the next day. He challenged me to answer questions asked by physicians and nurses and to research primary literature to support my answers. In return for my hard work, he always included me when physicians needed his help. I got to see traumas, cardioversions, infections, and toxicology cases. During that time, I learned not only about many medications and the pharmacodynamic interactions on the patient, but also about respect, empathy, and building relationships with your peers.

One of the last patients I saw as a student was a person who had been in a traumatic bicycle versus car accident where the biker was not wearing a helmet. He had flipped his bike and gone headfirst through the back windshield of the car. In the hectic trauma room, Brett was busy preparing medications to intubate and sedate the patient when the physician yelled out that they, also, wanted seizure prophylaxis and antibiotics for the operating room. In contrast to my first day, I quickly left the room and returned with the medications, prepared the doses, and had Brett double-check the products before giving them to the nurses. At that moment, I realized how much I had learned in 1 short month. I had gained confidence in myself, critical thinking skills, a passion for hospital pharmacy practice, and a mentor.

Now, as a newly practicing pharmacist, I hope to lead by example and become a mentor to students who spend time with me. I want to provide valuable and challenging experiences to help them grow as clinicians and gain confidence in themselves. Most importantly, I want to become an avenue of support as they continue through their careers in the same way my mentors continue to do for me.

Because of You

Amanda C. Chuk, Pharm.D., BCPS
Preceptor

*B*ecause of you. These words carry much meaning for the person who discovers that he or she helped someone else accomplish a goal. Within the field of pharmacy, one may hear such words uttered by a grateful patient who can now select appropriate over-the-counter medications because of a pharmacist's recommendation. Or the words may be said by the director of a hospital pharmacy department to the pharmacist who develops a cost-saving therapeutic interchange proposal. I want to share why those words were important to me during my practice as a clinical pharmacist specialist at an academic medical center.

In addition to my clinical duties in the adult intensive care unit, I serve as a preceptor for introductory and advanced pharmacy practice experiential (I/APPE) rotations through several schools of pharmacy. The introductory rotation during the early professional program years involves the students spending time in each area of our pharmacy department. James is one student who was scheduled to complete an IPPE at our hospital. Although James' school of pharmacy was quite a distance from our hospital, his parents lived in a nearby town. The availability of a rotation outside his school's immediate surroundings and the prospect of spending a month with family enticed him to come to our hospital for an IPPE rotation.

James was due to spend several days with me in the ICU during his rotation. On our first scheduled morning, a well-dressed young man came to my office, white coat and notepad in hand. His look conveyed a sense of professionalism and motivation. When I greeted James, I introduced myself and asked him about his career aspirations. He didn't hesitate before answering, "I want to work in retail."

Immediately, I knew it might be a challenge for me to hold James' attention in a hospital setting when his interest lay in community pharmacy. However, I gave him an overview of my job as a critical care pharmacist, and we walked to the ICU to join the team of physicians and medical students who had started to gather there. Rounds began, and in each patient's room, we stood at the bedside and listened to the physicians' presentations while hearing input from the nurses and respiratory therapists. As was my daily routine, I used the time to make therapeutic recommendations to the team to optimize the current or proposed medication plan. I took the opportunity to ask James about some of the medications with which he may have been familiar at that point in his training. After rounds were completed, he and I also reviewed the patients' home medications that were not continued upon admission to the ICU. This prompted a discussion regarding the reasons behind interruption in some therapies, and I highlighted the role a pharmacist can have in medication reconciliation across environments of care.

In the afternoon, while I worked on projects, James shadowed our other decentralized clinical pharmacists who work in the ICU and serve as sources of drug information for nurses while assisting prescribers with the selection and dosing of medications. James and I would meet to discuss the patient cases and new pieces of knowledge gained through his exposure to these critically ill patients. Some of the home medications that were not continued on the first day of the patient's ICU admission could be restarted safely and appropriately, and James assisted in the recommendations to the team to resume those therapies. We agreed that other home medications, lacking an obvious association with a current medical problem, were best left discontinued to avoid unnecessary medication therapy (we also agreed that we would ask the team to clarify the plan for those therapies before the patient's discharge from the ICU).

After this routine during the next few days, James developed a thorough approach to each new patient and constantly asked questions regarding the medications used. Although his therapeutic expertise was in its beginning stage, James identified medications that were similar to what he had seen in the retail setting. He then used his background knowledge to evaluate the pharmacy profiles of the ICU patients he followed, forming lists of opportunities for interventions and suggestions for change. I could sense that even in our few days together, James was beginning to expand his critical thinking skills. Through our question-and-answer sessions, his dedication was evident to me, and I was provided a look into the type of clinical pharmacist practitioner James would someday become. I would soon learn he was experiencing the same glimpse into his potential professional future in a hospital setting, a future much different from the one he had imagined for himself in retail pharmacy. The end of the week came quickly, and James was scheduled to spend the remainder of his rotation in different practice areas of our hospital pharmacy department.

One day at the end of the month, I walked into a shared office where our clinical pharmacy manager was speaking with James. When I asked him about the rest of his rotation, he said, "I changed my mind and want to work as a hospital pharmacist because of you." Thinking he meant you in a collective way to describe his experience in our hospital, I said how wonderful it was that our department was able to offer him such a positive introduction to hospital pharmacy. He smiled, shook his head, and repeated, "No, because of you," pointing his finger at me.

He went on to describe the role he was able to play in proactively recommending changes and additions to a patient's therapeutic plan. Until this time, his experience in community pharmacy practice had offered him examples of reactive interventions the pharmacist made regarding prescribed medications. He shared that he was excited at the prospect of applying his knowledge of pharmacy while assisting physicians in the development of treatment plans for patients in the hospital. He also said that joining the pharmacists alongside the physicians, nurses, and respiratory therapists in discussing each patient in the ICU showed him that the pharmacist is an integral member of the health care team.

Two years later, during his final year of professional training, James returned to our hospital and completed an advanced rotation with me as his preceptor in our critical care unit. He came armed with a more developed background in therapeutics and easily applied this knowledge to all aspects of care for ICU patients. Our discussions delved into not only ambulatory medicine but also critical care–specific therapies and disease-state management strategies. As I had come to expect from his earlier rotation, James continued to apply a comprehensive approach to each patient when reviewing and assessing the medication plan. Although I have since lost track of his whereabouts, I have no doubt that James is a confident and compassionate addition to the pharmacist workforce.

Serendipitously, what at first appeared to be simply a convenient location for an IPPE rotation was, instead, a turning point for James in his clinical training. Truthfully, I am unsure of the exact moment that led to this. James brought to the rotation an intrinsic enthusiasm for learning and recognition of the importance of patient-centered care. I share these attributes, and I was first attracted to join the staff of our department because of its commitment to implementing pharmacy teams in care areas throughout the hospital. Perhaps this pharmacy practice setting was unfamiliar to James and he was unaware of the contributions a pharmacist can make to the management of hospitalized patients. He claimed inspiration from the professional relationships that the pharmacist team of critical care staff and I maintain with other health care providers and the clinical pharmacy services we offer in the ICU. To discover that both the passion I have and the confidence I continue to build are outwardly apparent to others is rewarding news. However, I do not share this story as a boost to my own ego. James helped me see that among the many titles held by pharmacists (medication expert, patient counselor, technician manager, etc.), two of the most satisfying are preceptor and role model. I have learned that any interaction with a student is potentially a defining moment made possible *because of you.*

Precepting and Teaching Students for Success: Keep It Positive!

Peter Gal, Pharm.D.
Educator/Clinician

When I was in pharmacy school in the early 1970s, I often watched my professors' teaching approaches, thinking there must be a better way. So many times, we were asked to memorize material that the teachers could not memorize. They would read their notes as they wrote information or drew structures on the chalkboard. The message was obvious: this information is not even important enough for me to memorize correctly, but you must memorize it because I have the power to fail you. Then, the exams reflected the same meaningless, mind-numbing detail in ways sure to make you get much of the information wrong. Clerkship rotations were much better, but many preceptors were focused on impressing me with their knowledge and making sure I duly respected their importance and power. There was a tendency to play students against each other so that some would appear to be the best prepared and the smartest. However, all of this belied my belief that education could be demanding and fun and that colleagues could challenge and improve each other without problematic interpersonal interactions. Furthermore, because learning is a continuous process, with facts frequently changing and evolving, I believe it is important for students to integrate a process of continuous learning into their professional behavior.

When I became faculty, I naturally wanted to emulate the preceptors who I felt had taught me the most, even though many of these individuals could be quite intimidating. Although these preceptors enabled highly motivated students to reach their potential, they sometimes frustrated students with less ability. Like the preceptors, though, I, too, was a demanding teacher, and to some extent, I focused on and rewarded the students who were most accomplished.

However, parenthood changes you... When I had a son and he was old enough to play soccer, I started coaching. Although many parents yelled at their kids during the game, I realized that yelling made the kids stressed, frustrated, and reluctant to try innovative moves for fear of making a mistake. I included a silly drill in every practice to get the kids to laugh and made a point of encouraging the kids' creativity and freedom to select and run to open spaces, rewarding the players who ran to these spaces by getting the ball to them. I sat down with the parents and emphasized their need to say only positive things, and I made sure all the players got fair time to play. This creative, flowing, and fun style was beautiful to watch and great fun for the kids, and it got us many compliments from the referees who managed our games. The way players supported each other, encouraging one another to be creative, strengthened the personal relationships of the players and their families. When the state tournament came, these kids won each game by at least four goals, including the final, and other coaches, players, and referees praised our players for their cohesion and teamwork.

Because professional practice also requires a collaborative, cohesive, and open-minded approach, it seems reasonable to train students to develop these attitudes and integrate a more thoughtful approach into their practice. It also seemed reasonable to create a similar trusting environment in the classroom. To accomplish this, we needed to emphasize that students were entitled to express their opinions and state facts (correct or incorrect), with the confidence that they would not be negatively criticized, but rather, that discussion would be encouraged. The idea was that all students—the brilliant, the assertive, the shy, and the not so sure—could excel and learn to participate and that the whole would achieve far more than the sum of its parts. This experiment in the use of an overwhelmingly positive teaching approach benefited from the combination of three faculty teaching our seminar course. Two of us took opposite sides regarding the same facts, and the third took the middle road. Role modeling the idea that it is possible to interpret facts in different ways helped students recognize the possibility of legitimate differences in viewpoints. We did not add our opinions until all students had been given the opportunity to comment.

Over time, as we refined our positive approach, we noticed a gradual shift from a class where the star students clearly dominated the discussion, and the less confident or less accomplished students said little and made inferior presentations of cases or topics, to a class where each student's special value to the group was the focus. This past year, the class came closest to reaching our goals yet. We had students in the class who were in the top 10 percent and several who (by GPA) were in the bottom 10 percent. Despite this, each brought special perspectives that enriched the others. For example, the academically strongest students would challenge the selection of drug therapy on the basis of various published studies or bring up excellent critiques of the studies used to justify a therapy. Students less oriented toward analysis of the clinical literature would bring in humanistic issues often overlooked by the others. They would ask about patient preferences, previous patient experiences with drugs in a certain class, and economic or social barriers to patients getting the best therapy academically. When each group (reassured by our encouragement to state its position) confidently engaged in discussions and debates about patient preference versus best therapeutic option, the entire class benefited and grew. This worked so well that, this past year, two of us were recognized by students for teaching excellence. More important was the party the students gave for us at the end of the year to thank us for creating such a good learning experience. Our actual reward was watching how each student grew in self-confidence, professionalism, and comfort through professional debates with classmates.

Our teaching group had seen this evolving for years. Each year, we asked for critiques so that we could tweak the process and blend academic education with confidence building. This past year, the class differences were perhaps greater than most starting out. By the second half of the year, we noticed that the class seemed to plan a group dinner once a week. They encouraged and supported each other. They did what health professionals should do: "care for other people." They were comfortable admitting limitations and asking advice from others without the fear of negative connotations. In addition, they freely shared opinions that might be useful to their colleagues and, more importantly, the patients they would one day serve. In my opinion, people who behave this way with each other become the best health care providers.

Things I Learned During My Psychiatric Pharmacy Rotation: A Daily Diary by "Pharmacy Student"

Brooke D. Butler, Pharm.D.
Resident

William Klugh Kennedy, Pharm.D., BCPP, FASHP
Educator

Things I learned on **Day 1** of my Psych rotation: (1) Pillowcases are acceptable fashion accessories on a psych ward. (2) If you do not understand random babble: smile, nod, and say "Yes, sir" or "Yes, ma'am." (3) Do like Forrest Gump and wear comfortable shoes.

Things I learned on **Day 2** of my Psych rotation: (1) When the curtain is drawn, it is drawn for a reason. Do not enter, or you will likely see something unpleasant. (2) The brown mystery thing on the floor might be a cookie. Don't always assume the worst. (3) Do not, I repeat, do not fall out of a golf cart and damage your frontal lobe.

Things I learned on **Day 3** of my Psych rotation: (1) All the names of the benzodiazepines sound the same when they are said by someone with no teeth. (2) Hospital gowns do not cover nearly enough, and 75-year-old testicles are incredibly ugly.

Things I learned on **Day 4** of my Psych rotation: (1) If you give orange juice to an angry old man with schizophrenia, he will likely throw it at you. (2) The policeman guarding the arrestee's room does not like it when you sing "I Fought the Law" to him.

Things I learned on **Day 5** of my Psych rotation: (1) When you have dementia, you *do* still care what color shoes you wear that day, contrary to this pharmacy student's expectations. (2) Surprisingly, 86-year-old women are capable of kicking out reinforced windows.

Things I learned on **Day 6** of my Psych rotation: (1) Cafeteria oatmeal cookies are "very yummy." (2) Lorazepam makes people stop yelling at you.

Things I learned on **Day 7** of my Psych rotation: (1) If you don't want to talk to your doctor, fake sleep. However, if you *are* playing possum, do not open one eye to see if they are still there. (2) Ink stains are the enemy of lab coats. Clicker pens are convenient and much more white coat–friendly. (3) Apparently, when you've been institutionalized for a month, all you can think about is sex, booze, and cigarettes.

Things I learned on **Day 8** of my Psych rotation: (1) Having only three follow-ups and no new patients is *awesome* because it means you get done at *3* p.m. instead of *7* p.m. (2) No matter how bad it gets, a 6-inch steak knife to the abdomen is *not* the answer.

Things I learned on **Day 9** of my Psych rotation: (1) Most patients are fairly private, but every now and then, you get the rare ones that want to talk about their bowel habits. Today, I hit the jackpot. (2) Nurses seriously have the hardest jobs at the hospital. They do and see lots of unpleasant things; major kudos to them.

Things I learned on **Day 10** of my Psych rotation: (1) Avoid intentionally angering your next-door neighbor. If you do, there is a chance she will hit you in the face with a hammer. (2) If you *do* decide to kill yourself, God forbid, do not make your own gun. You will fail…, and it will suck.

Things I learned on **Day 11** of my Psych rotation: (1) Even though I don't *want* to know your sexual history, I am still required to ask. Believe me; I could go my whole life without knowing how many male *and* female partners you've had. (2) There will be times when holding your breath is just not enough.

Things I learned on **Day 12** of my Psych rotation: (1) Doctors will answer to "Detective," too, so don't feel bad if you are confused. (2) Pulling out your indwelling catheter is *not* the best plan. You might be on opioids and haloperidol today, but tomorrow, your junk is gonna hurt.

Things I learned on **Day 13** of my Psych rotation: (1) The "voices" will sometimes choose you to be the one that gets beat up. (2) You don't know what awkward feels like until your floridly schizophrenic patient decides to start flirting with you. (3) If you are ever hospitalized and you get tired of your IV line, chew through it. It *can* be done—I've seen it.

Things I learned on **Day 14** of my Psych rotation: (1) Prepare yourself in advance for what may come out of a patient's duffle bag: possibly sharp objects or living things. (2) When asking bipolar patients about their hobbies, do not be surprised when they say, "I like to have sex." (3) The Earth is going to be destroyed because Pluto has come out of its orbit and is causing a cosmic gravitational imbalance.

Things I learned on **Day 15** of my Psych rotation: (1) Don't take away an old lady's salt because she will put you on her "shit-list." (2) The Chang brothers monopolize the lawnmower industry and ruined one of my patient's lives. They also invented cell phones that give you brain cancer. Shame on them!

Things I learned on **Day 16** of my Psych rotation: (1) Buy extra virgin olive oil instead of ibuprofen to cure your headaches. The patient writing an algorithm on a scrap of paper to correct his lithium level told me this, so it must be true. (2) Drug companies are evil and out to steal our souls. (I already knew this…, but thanks for pointing it out.)

Things I learned on **Day 17** of my Psych rotation: (1) I wear too much eyeliner. (2) I need to button my blouse. (3) I didn't put on enough rouge this morning…, and apparently, my natural color is "pale."

Things I learned on **Day 18** of my Psych rotation: (1) Angry Birds to pass the time in the emergency department. (2) Don't make eye contact with the manic patient. If you do, it will result in a 15-minute tirade about how you doctors don't know a damn thing.

Things I learned on **Day 19** of my Psych rotation: (1) The elevator in behavioral medicine is absolutely, without a doubt, the slowest elevator in existence. I'm pretty sure it was the first one ever invented by Mr. Otis. (2) Use tongs to pick up the biscuit in the breakfast tray or the cafeteria lady will yell at you. (3) Dr. Farrer has beautiful sable-brown eyelashes that most [78-year-old] women would die for.

Things I learned on **Day 20** of my Psych rotation: (1) Flu shot by blonde nurse = inability to move arm for 2 days. (2) Beards may contribute to poor personal hygiene...and result in treasure hunts!

Things I learned on **Day 21** of my Psych rotation: (1) *Do not* look in the trash cans. (2) When the schizophrenic patient is looking at the ceiling, don't assume he or she is just acting bizarre. There may be something up there...like a roach.

Things I learned on **Day 22** of my Psych rotation: (1) The students' lounge has a button beside the door that you have to push to get out. It is very upsetting. (2) Vomit creates new colors that not even God has seen before.

Things I learned on **Days 23** and **24** of my Psych rotation: (1) Mental illness is real. Just like coronary artery disease, diabetes, and cancer.... Patients suffering from mental illness deserve the same kind of respect and treatment as any other ailing individual. (2) Do not fear these people; just be careful (e.g., the agitated geriatric woman). Positive energy will get you everywhere. (3) Thank God every day that you were blessed with some kind of sanity. While we all have a little bit of "craziness" as part of our individuality, some people have to live with a monster inside them. Be grateful it isn't you.

When selecting rotations for my advanced pharmacy practice experience (APPE), I knew from the very beginning I wanted psychiatry for my specialty rotation. Many of my friends and fellow students were curious as to why I was so interested in spending my days in a psychiatric facility with the scary and sad mentally ill. I always did my best to explain. My grandfather, an advocate and counselor for the mentally ill, always said that the human brain is "the last frontier" of medicine. There is so much we don't know and have yet to learn about what exactly is inside that semisolid grey matter that makes us who we are as individuals. What little we do know regarding mental illness can be disheartening, yet fascinating, and there is an immediate, overwhelming need to further our understanding.

The five weeks that I spent at Memorial Hospital during my APPE were intense yet enjoyable ones. It's not that seeing human suffering was an easy or pleasant experience. It is one of the hardest things I've ever endured. There were times when I had to look away, so the patient would not see the tears forming in my eyes. In the evening, I would find myself at home, long after my day at the hospital had ended, thinking about the people I had encountered that day, searching the literature for answers or at least options. It was more often than not that God heard my patients' names in my nightly prayers.

So what, you may ask, is enjoyable about psychiatry? Why should I, as a pharmacy student, want to spend five weeks caring for the mentally ill? I will give you the answer. Because of the look of hopelessness in the eyes of my patient who just couldn't find a reason not to stab himself with that steak knife. Because of the sincere next-day apology from the schizophrenic man who threw his orange juice at me, and knowing, that deep down, it wasn't really him who would do such a thing. Because of the overwhelming gratitude displayed by my little ninja attack lady when I brought her a sack of romance novels and a $2 pair of reading glasses. Because of my mother, who is bipolar type I, my hero and my best friend. For it is these people, and many more, who have touched and inspired me to complete this PGY-1 residency and go on to become a psychiatric pharmacist.

No cure exists for the people I encountered during my rotation on the behavioral medicine service. There is no cure for my mother. However, there are people like you, and like me, with the capability, education, and motivation to help these people; to make a difference in their lives. Together, we can continue to research, hope and pray, endure the worse, remember the best... and laugh at the absurd.

Pharmacy Prospects

Shaping the Future

*We are made wise not by the recollection of
our past, but by the responsibility for our future.*

George Bernard Shaw

*If education is always to be conceived along the
same antiquated lines of a mere transmission
of knowledge, there is little to be hoped from
it in the bettering of man's future. For what
is the use of transmitting knowledge if the
individual's total development lags behind?*

Maria Montessori

Balancing Competing Patient Care Philosophies During Ambulatory Care APPEs

Jeffrey M. Brewer, Pharm.D.
Preceptor

Paul Denvir, Ph.D.
Researcher

"Good Morning. Welcome to my family medicine advanced pharmacy practice experience (APPE). During this module, we will explore the role of interpersonal communication in the profession of pharmacy, the pharmacist provider philosophy, and focus on the interaction between patients and providers. Which modules have you completed this year?"

An eager-looking student obliged: "Well, on module A, I was at my community rotation. This was very similar to my work experience. I spent the past 3 years at a community pharmacy in town. Module B was my institutional rotation for 12 weeks. I spent most of my time in the pharmacy and learned how to make IVs, filled the robot, checked the cart, and processed orders up on the patient floors. During module C, I worked in the drug information unit of a pharmaceutical company. That was interesting; I found the interaction with the callers stimulating. I love to learn new things and research medication information. Now I am here with you on module D." As he spoke, I found myself wondering whether he had experienced the patient-focused philosophy before my module.

When he finished, I prompted him again: "Sounds like you've experienced many of the core areas where pharmacists practice. What do you hope to gain from my experience?"

This time, he took longer to answer. It is not uncommon for students to be stumped by this question. He had chosen his modules 8 months earlier, and his thought process could have been very different now that he had finished half of his APPEs. After an internal dialogue, he said, "I heard this was a challenging rotation where I would use my customer service and counseling skills. I see the ups and downs of community pharmacy, and I love helping people. I am hoping to become more confident in my interaction with customers and physicians." At this point, I was getting nervous. The terminology he used was typical of more product-focused pharmacists, very different from the patient-focused philosophy I try to practice and teach.

Sensing a budding conflict, I focused on my terminology and expectations. "You will definitely be challenged on this experience. I expect you to function as a pharmacy provider in this setting. That means you will be a problem solver regarding the medication-related problems that you identify. In this setting, you will never be the final decision-maker. However, I expect you to bring a fully formed plan to the discussion after every patient interaction. The first part of your experience will be focused on the collection and organization of patient information. Once you are comfortable with the information you have organized, you will need to make an accurate, evidence-based assessment. Then, we will focus on committing to a plan and implementing it with the patient's medical provider."

It was clear from his body language that this philosophy and approach to practice was not in his professional comfort zone. With obvious reluctance, he responded with a fairly insightful critique of himself. "I did well on my SOAP notes in class, and I feel confident that I can organize the data. The areas that I am weakest in are assessment, plan, and convincing the medical providers to take my recommendation." It was good to hear that he had experience with self-evaluation and insight. This is not a common skill in students. However, at this point, I was confident that I needed to review the basics of direct patient care and delve into his patient care philosophy.

Two Weeks Later...
We were sitting in the clinic mid-morning, and I offered him a challenge: "I can see that you are getting a feel for the patient population here. We saw several complex patients this morning, and there are a couple of patients whom we have not yet discussed. Why don't you present one of them? I felt like you were uncomfortable with what I was asking you to do."

Slightly agitated, the student clarified: "I was not uncomfortable, I just don't see the application of some of the tasks that we are doing here. They seem to be the doctor's job. I am connecting with the patients and identifying many of their drug-related problems. The medication and allergy list was complete, and I professionally conveyed that to the provider."

At this point, I could clearly see that our practice philosophies were going to be antagonistic. Trying to keep my cool, I led with the positives: "Okay. I liked your prioritization of the problems that you addressed on the last two patients. When we talked about assessment and plan last week, we discussed taking ownership of the patient in front of you. As the pharmacist provider at this site, you should collect pertinent data, organize it to tell a story, and then assess and plan for the necessary changes that will help patients achieve their goals. I also noticed that you shied away from triaging the patient's complaint and did not commit to a plan of action. Specifically, it was important to do a symptom analysis on the patient's chief concern. One reason was to better inform you about whether the issue could be triaged to the OTC aisle, the provider's office, or the emergency room. This also serves to let the patient know you are listening. Additionally, the next step in your relationship with the provider team is at the colleague level. When you brought solutions to the patient's disease and medication-related problems to the medical provider, you became more valuable to the health care team. Otherwise, you are no different from any other staff member who collected data for the provider to think about. Help me understand why this piece was difficult for you."

The student was now openly frustrated. He tersely responded: "I understand what you are saying about being a pharmacy provider. However, this is not what I was trained to do and what I will be doing when I graduate. The supervisor from my community job says that when I graduate, I will need to focus on meeting my performance goals and spend less time on things that I have no control over."

As I drove home that night, I kept coming back to that familiar phrase in my mind: "This is not what I'll be doing when I graduate." It certainly wasn't the first time I had heard a student say it. Honestly, I hear that on my APPE several times a year. What I wondered was, how could two people in the same profession have such different ideas about where the profession is going? I'd like to share my thoughts.

There are two philosophies of practice that are prevalent in the profession of pharmacy today. These philosophies are on a continuum and represent how we think about patients and how we prioritize our days. Both philosophies can be found in new and seasoned pharmacists as well as in all areas of pharmacy practice. The first is a product-based philosophy. In this philosophy, the pharmacist sees him- or herself as the final step in the medication use process. He or she provides the correct medication to the correct patient. This has been pharmacy's core business for a long time and is the most recognized function that pharmacists provide. The second is a patient-based philosophy. In that philosophy, the pharmacist sees him- or herself as integral to the entire medication use process. With others in the health care team, the pharmacist designs the correct medication therapy to treat the correct patient. Regardless of access to the full medical record, the pharmacist reviews all the available data (medical record, patient, caregiver) and monitors the patient to ensure safe and effective medication therapy usage.

In the ambulatory care APPE, this clash of philosophies can be extreme for students who have solidified a product-based philosophy. One setting for the ambulatory care APPE is a private physician office. Practicing pharmacy in this setting is characterized by reviewing the patient's medication and medical history, taking responsibility for and triaging the patient's health care needs, and collaborating with providers on therapy decisions. The pharmacy student who has solidified a product-based philosophy can be overwhelmed with the patient-based philosophy, the process involved in taking responsibility for the patient's health, and communicating complex therapeutic decisions. Many times, these students effectively pare down their patient care role in an attempt to adjudicate their professional philosophy with what they view as the pharmacist's role. They are efficient with collecting data and counseling on the usage of specific medications. These actions frequently meet the expectations of the provider. However, these students are short-changing their training and potential synergistic collaboration with the provider when they do not fully work up a comprehensive plan for a drug-related problem or triage a new patient complaint.

The discrepancy between the potential future taught by patient-focused preceptors and the current reality of the business of pharmacy can be confusing for students. It is this friction between the business of pharmacy and the profession of pharmacy that, in many ways, defines the level of frustration in pharmacy students and burnout in practicing pharmacists. With experience and efficiency, our patient-focused preceptors can help students bridge this intersection between business interests and professional interests. More importantly, we need to help them recognize where they are on the patient-focused continuum. This discussion will help them identify their goal as well as envision a future where the patient's needs are considered equal to or above business interests. Optimally, the business interests and professional interests intersect in the patient-focused philosophy.

Successful pharmacy students are those who are able to balance their professional duties to the patient with the business requirement of their setting. The majority of pharmacy practice areas require a seamless melding of the product- and patient-focused philosophies. Therefore, the two biggest challenges for patient-focused preceptors are the alignment of a student's philosophy with the worksite philosophy and the discussion of expectations when barriers to this philosophy exist.

Six Weeks Later...

As I complete his final evaluation, I reflect on the conflict of the past 6 weeks and consider a place for both opinions. He got high marks on identifying and collecting the data, interacting with the patients, and his professional approach to the physician office. He got low marks for his inability to pull together an in-depth plan for the patient as well as his implementation of that plan with the providers. In many ways, this is a function of his philosophy—the belief that his job ended when the correct medication was delivered to the correct patient. Ultimately, I believe he will be unprepared for the role of the pharmacist provider that the profession of pharmacy is headed for and, in some states and settings, already encountering.

Clinical Pharmacists Are Everywhere

Kayce M. Shealy, Pharm.D., BCPS
Educator/Clinician

I completed a community practice residency after pharmacy school because I am drawn to the community sector. I feel that there is a huge need for pharmacists in community settings to provide quality care to a wide variety of patients. The community setting, to me, can be considered the frontline of care. Patients spend more time in the community than in any other health care arena, and I feel it is our responsibility to help keep them there. In this setting, though, I feel that I often have to prove I am a competent clinician, not only to other health care providers but also to my colleagues and my students.

As I prepared for my day in the physicians' office where I currently practice, a student entered my office seeking research opportunities. I was a little caught by surprise—she is a first-year, first-semester student—and what in the world does she know about research in pharmacy practice? As I listened to her intentions, interests, and plans for the next couple of years, I found myself extremely proud that we are instilling a sense of scholarship in our students early on. Then she said it: "I know that I definitely want to be a clinical pharmacist, not work in the community."

Now, maybe I was not in the best of moods before she entered my office. I was frustrated with students for asking the same questions over and over again in class. I was frustrated because I wasn't able to devote as much time to developing my practice site as my colleagues did because of my high teaching load, and somehow, our e-mail server had randomly started sending e-mails to the junk folder. Nonetheless, her statement felt like a punch in the stomach. I felt as if I had been validating myself and my skills to everyone lately. I am a board-certified pharmacotherapy specialist; I am residency-trained; I have demonstrated scholarship; I have demonstrated ability to perform patient care. I realize that I am a new practitioner and new clinical faculty member, but what more do I have to do to earn respect?

I interrupted her as she continued to talk about her potential research interests. I asked, "What do you mean when you say *clinical?*" Her response: "Working in a hospital." Then, I inquired, "What about a hospital makes a clinical pharmacist?" and "Why are pharmacists who work in a community not considered clinical?" She replied to my questions by saying that interacting with other health care providers, making recommendations about a patient's medication regimen and providing direct patient care, wearing a long white coat, and obtaining specialty certification would classify a pharmacist as *clinical.*

"OK," I said, "I am getting ready to go to the clinic and see patients with physicians in my long white coat. Behind my name is *Pharm.D., BCPS*, the same as every other faculty member in this department. Some of my duties in the clinic are to talk with patients about their diseases like diabetes and heart failure, educate them about drug therapy, tell them why it is important, and suggest recommendations to optimize therapy to the patient's physician such as adding metformin or increasing lisinopril. I document any interventions I may have made and then follow up with the patients to determine if the therapy or intervention is effective. When I am in the pharmacy, I address medication adherence, perform medication therapy management, and recommend any changes to the patient's primary provider to improve the patient's care. I also check patients' blood pressure, blood glucose, and cholesterol; I provide immunizations and have prescriptive authority for the influenza vaccine. One of my colleagues down the hall meets with patients and actually makes necessary therapy changes herself because she has a collaborative agreement with the provider to do so. She doesn't practice in a hospital, though. Is any of that *clinical*, in your opinion?"

I am sure that she did not see this coming. An innocent gesture to talk about research possibilities for the future turned into a 20-minute soapbox rant on clinical pharmacy. At the conclusion of my lecture, the student looked overwhelmed, and she was taken aback. Then, she said, "Well, I never thought about it like that. Maybe clinical pharmacists are everywhere, not just a hospital." *Point for me*, I thought.

I continue to be very excited about the expanding roles and potential for clinical pharmacists in every setting. Competent, caring, capable, and professional pharmacists are needed everywhere, from the hospital to the health department to the retail pharmacy on the corner. Our training equips us with the skills and knowledge to be *clinical*; it just has to be applied in our practice. As health care reform evolves and more focus is placed on quality and prevention, clinical pharmacists in every setting will be needed to provide pharmaceutical care to help improve patient outcomes while decreasing costs. I hope we can instill in student pharmacists that clinical pharmacy doesn't fit into a box and is not one-size-fits-all.

Respected Colleague

Gary Milavetz, Pharm.D., B.S.
Researcher/Educator/Clinician

S tarting a professional career is challenging and stressful, but it can be very rewarding. Professional acceptance is a key ingredient in being part of a health care team. I was comfortable with both my knowledge base and my clinical skills. More importantly, I had the tools to find the answers to what I didn't know and enough experience to guide judgment calls when no clear answer could be found. However, there was always this nagging doubt whether I was truly accepted as a member of the Pediatric Allergy Clinic care team. Even though my recommendations were implemented and I was included in all team activities from radiology rounds (where I couldn't read an image, but learned from it) to coffee breaks and care conferences, I still wondered about my role on the team. Trust, respect, and acceptance occur in small positive steps punctuated by occasional glints of insight gained in retrospection.

After several years of participating in inpatient rounds and outpatient clinics and of writing research proposals including protocols, my value among my physician colleagues was built and appreciated. Soon, they were introducing me as "Dr. Milavetz, our clinical pharmacist." It continued to develop to the point one day that I overheard the Pediatric Allergy/Pulmonary Division Chair telling one of the pediatric residents in training to take theophylline dosing and level adjustment recommendations only from the physicians or clinical pharmacist on the service. Wow! So there I was, 1 of about 70 pharmacists in the institution at the time, and the Pediatric Allergy/Pulmonary Division Chair instructed the pediatric residents to listen to me!

Any last self-doubt about my role on the team was completely alleviated one late fall day in clinic. After a long and busy clinic, one of the faculty physicians and I were standing in the treatment room, finishing up paperwork. All the other health care providers in clinic that day had either left for the day or gone back to their offices to complete notes and check messages. We reviewed a couple of interesting findings from the patients seen and discussed the pros and cons of a treatment choice for one patient. We made some small talk about the fall season and the preparations for winter, including vaccinations for our clinic patients. He asked if I had received an influenza vaccination this year. When I responded yes, he asked who administered it. I told him one of the clinic nurses, as that was the usual practice in our clinic at the time. Although this event occurred about 10 years before immunizations were included in professional practice regulations, many advanced practice pharmacists were skilled in drawing blood for pharmacokinetic analysis and a few, including myself, were experienced in giving injections as a routine part of their patient care. Looking directly at me, he said, "Why don't you give me a flu shot now?" Although I smiled at him and said "sure," a wave of apprehension fell over me, and I started to sweat. Not the hot temperature or exertion kind, but the autonomic kind when you feel particularly stressed. I told myself to "maintain homeostasis" while feeling slightly lightheaded. Although I had given dozens of subcutaneous injections in the past to patients, including to several patients who were unwilling, I had never given one to "the boss"! He started to roll up his sleeve while I obtained the pre-loaded syringe from the refrigerator. I rolled it between my hands to mix and warm it. The movement helped dissipate the light-headedness and refocus my attention. I prepped the skin on his arm, administered the injection, and put a bandage on it. He matter-of-factly said "thanks" and walked away. There was no drama for him or from him during the ordeal.

As his footsteps on the floor receded, I pumped a fist in the air, mouthed a silent "yes," and smiled broadly. I breathed a sigh of relief that everything went well and realized he had just given me one of the highest compliments of trust. I now knew without a doubt that I was truly respected as a colleague. Trust and team acceptance among health professionals occur over time with shared experiences. Working with this group of health care professionals through the Pediatric Allergy/Pulmonary Clinic has been very positive and full of opportunities for advancing my career. With patience and perseverance, this pharmacist was able to become an integral member of the Pediatric Allergy Clinic care team, diminishing any self-doubts about trust, respect, and acceptance.

Patient Champion

Margie Padilla, Pharm.D., CDE
Clinician

Often, it is difficult to articulate and fully grasp the work of a clinical pharmacist. I find myself consistently promoting my services. In fact, it has become part of my daily routine. Yet I never imagined I would find a patient advocating for my services. This gentleman transcended barriers that I'd been struggling and working through in the past couple of years at my clinic. He sought my assistance with his disease state, but in reality, he helped me overcome provider adversity and come to a better understanding of interprofessional care.

My clinic provides culturally appropriate services in English and Spanish and uses educators and *promotoras* (lay workers) in disease prevention and education. Because our community is mostly Hispanic, many unique issues need to be addressed—for example, the fear of insulin, which is perceived as a death sentence; patients equate it to cancer. We also counsel patients on issues such as medications purchased in Mexico and the use of herbal products. I work closely with a physician champion, Dr. Alvarado, who is supportive of the culturally appropriate services we extend to his patients. This support has been vital in the start-up and expansion of clinical pharmacy services.

Dr. Alvarado strongly believes patient outcomes will improve if we work together and address medication issues.

Currently, I am able to manage most chronic diseases under a collaborative agreement. In the past year, we have been able to prescribe dangerous drugs (non-narcotics) because of recent changes in our state laws. With the advocacy of Dr. Alvarado, the Chief Clinical Officer of our federally qualified community health center, we have gained support from other providers such as nurse practitioners, physician assistants, counselors, health educators, promotoras, and a psychiatrist. For the past couple of years, we have been working toward obtaining support from some of our physician colleagues, with slow results. In the past few months, I've been working diligently at proving our value in patient care with a couple of our physicians, who do not see the benefit in the clinical services we provide. As a result, Dr. Maldonado, one of my physician colleagues, placed a block on his patients from consulting with me for their disease state management needs. Once I visited with his patients, I was unable to reschedule that patient for a follow-up in my clinic. It was very discouraging. It was a patient champion who helped change his mind.

Before the block in my schedule, Mr. Rodriguez, one of Dr. Maldonado's patients, was scheduled for a diabetes follow-up. He had been in my care for some time. In the past year, he had lost control of his diabetes. His HGA1C had increased to about 13%. His insulin regimen had also changed. He was no longer on his premixed Novolin 70/30 regimen, the insulin of choice on our clinic formulary. Uninsured and unable to qualify for Medicare/Medicaid, he was switched to an insulin regimen that consisted of Lantus and NovoLog, agents provided through our medication assistance program. Dr. Maldonado had made the change and referred him out for a consult with an endocrinologist. Mr. Rodriguez kept his visit and found that the specialist did not address his more immediate concerns with his diabetes. Mr. Rodriguez spent over $600 on what he felt was a lecture and nutritional counseling. The endocrinologist had not addressed his regimen or his blood sugar levels. He was extremely disappointed with the outcome of this visit and with Dr. Maldonado. The physician, he felt, had lost faith in his ability to make changes. Not only was his diabetes uncontrolled, but he had also incurred more debt. He wanted my assistance in controlling his blood sugar levels. He knew he was controlled, before this change, with my help. His next appointment with Dr. Maldonado was scheduled in 3 months, and he wanted to prove that he could control his sugars with my assistance. I agreed to help him establish control, not knowing, at this point, about the block in my schedule.

I met with Mr. Rodriguez every 2–3 weeks. He worked on his blood sugar control by eating better, exercising daily, and adhering to his medication changes. I was also able to address the lack of access to his NovoLog by using the medication assistance program. In the meantime, I was able to provide NovoLog samples until they arrived in the pharmacy. This helped address access and discontinuation of his insulin. I was able to better understand why he had lost control in the first place. In combination with his discontinuation of NovoLog, he was injecting his insulin at the wrong time. Using his blood sugar log, we were able to identify these areas of concern, and we worked through them. His incorrect timing of insulin created a cycle of frequent low blood sugars between meals and high sugars before going to bed. This led to a cycle of uncontrolled sugars and self-decrease of insulin dose. Eventually, with the proper education on timing, we realized that he did better with a regimen that consisted of a split dose of Lantus in the morning and evening. He continued to take his NovoLog three times a day before meals. Once this regimen was set in place, his sugars slowly began to drop, and he finally reached a steady decline in blood sugar levels. This new regimen stopped his frequent symptoms of hypoglycemia. Fortunately, this happened before his scheduled visit with Dr. Maldonado. It was perfect timing because this was the last visit I was able to schedule. This is when I became aware of the scheduling block. Despite the scheduling obstacle, I flagged Dr. Maldonado in the electronic medical records and thanked him for the opportunity and trust in managing his patients. I was able to send a quick note on the status of Mr. Rodriguez.

To my surprise, a couple of weeks later, I saw that I had Mr. Rodriguez on my schedule for a follow-up appointment for his diabetes. I did not realize that my visit with him was after his visit with his primary care physician. As I walked into the visit, he greeted me, saying, "I have something to tell you. I had a huge talk and disagreement with my doctor." His news concerned me, as I thought this would really sever my relationship with the physician with whom I had been working extremely hard to build good rapport. Mr. Rodriguez explained that Dr. Maldonado was very upset with him for not following up with the endocrinologist he had been referred to earlier. He was also upset because Mr. Rodriguez did not follow his instructions. However, Mr. Rodriguez informed him that he had returned to my service because he had achieved prior control of his blood sugar levels when I was managing his diabetes. Dr. Maldonado told him, "But she is just a pharmacist." I could not believe how my patient responded to this statement: *"What does that matter? It's ultimately about providing the best care on my behalf. It's not about who is higher than the other. It's about what we both can do together."*

The patient told Dr. Maldonado that he was disappointed in his giving up on him and quickly referring him out. The physician did not attempt to determine and resolve the patient's loss of control. He was quick to make a referral. He did not take into consideration that Mr. Rodriguez could not afford those types of services. The patient went on to say that, he thought the clinic was there to help prevent this from happening. The physician has a great resource for controlling diabetes, and he did not use it. Although the patient was disappointed in his provider, he did not want to leave his services. He just wanted to be heard. He told his physician that he wanted to continue to see me for his diabetes management. When Mr. Rodriguez showed him the improvement in his glucose level, the physician did not know what to do with the information. Dr. Maldonado said, "I will continue to let you see her. If you lose control, then it's your fault."

Dr. Maldonado lifted the block not only on this patient but also on all of his patients. Currently, he continues to allow me to see his patients. I continue to work and communicate with him regarding decisions and care of his patients. It will take some time and patience before he truly understands my role. This will always be an area of challenge as a clinical pharmacist, but I will continue to move forward in all of my efforts to educate and communicate.

The patient revealed a great perspective. Credentials are important. The type of care and results we provide trump credentials. Mr. Rodriguez wanted us to work together for his behalf. He did not want us to lose faith in his ability to do his part. He had many financial and emotional obstacles that required a creative approach to his care. He believed in himself and wanted us to do the same.

Mr. Rodriguez's determination created a change in the perception of patient care. He was a key player in the way care should be provided: as a collaborative effort. Sometimes, to fully understand patients' needs, we as providers need to listen more carefully to their stories. Like me, you will one day be surprised to find a patient advocating for your services.

The Importance of Relationships Among Health Care Providers

Kristi Kelley, Pharm.D., BCPS, CDE
Clinician/Preceptor

I will never forget my home phone ringing on a random Thursday in April. At the time, we did not have caller ID, so I was surprised when I recognized the caller as one of the physicians from the private practice group where I worked. He said, "Isn't Johnny one of your rotation students?" I said yes, fearful of where the conversation was going. He proceeded to tell me that Johnny had presented a prescription for a controlled substance at the pharmacy that night and that it was written in such a way that the pharmacist became suspicious, resulting in a call to the local authorities and the arrest of the student. I really do not remember all the details of our conversation, but I do remember my horror over the situation. I remember feeling numb, just not knowing how to respond. By nature, I tend to apologize for things that are not within my control, so I know I apologized repeatedly. I remember the seasoned physician reassuring me that although he was frustrated, even angry, with the student, he was not angry with me. Although I felt horrible about the situation, I remember feeling reassured because of the way the physician handled our conversation. Even though I dreaded going to the clinic the next morning, I had no doubt where I stood in my professional relationship with that physician after the phone call.

Needless to say, however, that Thursday night was not restful as I replayed my phone conversation with the physician in my head over and over again regarding Johnny. I continued to think about my last interactions with my student before we had finished rotations for the day, wondering if something had been different and I just had not noticed. It was certainly easy to second-guess every aspect of my interactions with the student for the past 7 weeks.

Although the next morning in the clinic was not easy, the physician and staff directly affected were steadfast in their interactions with me. Regrouping on what we, a pharmacist and pharmacy students, did in clinic, my student's lapse ended up being a positive experience. It provided the entire clinic staff a chance to carefully examine every process involving student interactions in clinic—exposure to patients, medical records, sample medications, prescription pads, and provider identification numbers.

As a young pharmacist early in my career, this event truly could have been devastating to me and could have resulted in the site's closing its doors to the school with which I was affiliated. I was fortunate that this incident did not define my career as a pharmacist in a negative way. Nor did it end my position at the clinic. Although my career has been influenced by this event, I have often thought about why this incident resulted in largely positive, rather than negative, outcomes. Although I know there are many reasons for this, I think the professional and ethical relationship that had been established between the other health care providers and staff in the clinic and me, which was lived out every day in the clinic, was the main reason this event ended positively. I feel very fortunate that I was in a clinic full of supportive people who, despite witnessing a lapse in integrity by my student, never seemed to question my own integrity.

The stolen prescription incident has reminded me of the importance of establishing and maintaining professional relationships with those with whom you work on a daily basis. I have also realized that it is important to model professional relationships for students and engage them in these relationships whenever possible.

Work and Family—Family and Work

John E. Murphy, Pharm.D., BSPharm
Educator

Read a story, please, Dad.

I can't now, son; have to rest and collect my thoughts.

Let's go on the boat, Dad.

*Can't now, son, have to work this weekend—I'm on call—
maybe next week.*

I love that boy. From the moment we received the blood test results, I knew it was going to be great to have a child. Five years ago, you couldn't have made me believe I would have kids. Too hedonistic. Now there are two. When delivered, he looked a bit like E.T., but he was the cutest baby I had ever seen. He turned slightly blue, which was worrisome, but came out of it while lying on Mom's tummy.

I have fears of something happening to him—don't know how I could handle it. When he first came home, I would wish he would stop crying at night. When he did, I worried that he was no longer breathing. He said "Daddy" first, probably because I coached him from day 1.

He's growing up now, almost 2 years old. It seems too fast, but it is fun to be able to hold conversations with him. The problem lies in finding the time to do it. What with teaching, consult service, committees, organizations, speaking engagements, research, writing, etc.— the quest for money and fame. He learned to talk on the phone while I was gone for a 17-day stretch—necessity, I guess. What is the balance? Will I be a better father if I get an 8-to-5 job and possibly hate it, or will he be proud of my accomplishments (a legend in my own mind) and happy with the time we spend together? I wish days had 36 hours in them. Why don't teachers make enough money to be able to work just one job and stay above the poverty level? The Dean says you have to move to get a better salary (a hint?). It doesn't seem quite right.

My boy loves me. Sometimes I wonder how. The 10- to 12-hour days and persistent on-call schedule. Coming home tired and occasionally irritable.

The other day my grandparents were in town, and Grandpa was out swinging my son in the backyard. I was on the porch reading an article, laying back, and listening to the television. I heard my boy talking to Grandpa. Then he saw me through the window and said "I love you, Dad," several times, repeating it each time I told him of my love. Maybe things are working out all right. My boy loves me, and that's as good as anything else in my mind.

The Busy Cycle

Ricky Ogden, Pharm.D., BCPS
Clinician

A dangerous cycle has been developing for the past 10 years in the pharmacy profession. Allow a brief description of a hypothetical clinical pharmacist's day. The desk phone is ringing almost continuously, and the pager is buzzing like an angry hornet. Two project deadlines are looming, and none of your co-investigators will call/e-mail back. Ironically, though, everyone else who needs something from you decides to e-mail you right now, urgently. Patients are complaining about their medications, which obviously must be the fault of the pharmacy. Your pharmacy student is sputtering about why her journal club is not done, and your pharmacy resident has not sent slides to you for tomorrow's presentation, despite your many requests to him. This dangerous decade-long phenomenon may be called the "Busy Cycle" concept.

Does this hypothetical day sound familiar? This describes the typical clinical pharmacist in today's deadline-riddled, frantic-paced realm, where we practice. If not everyone has at least 24 hours of work to try to cram into a 10-hour day, then the delusional self-perceptions of inadequacy begin to creep into the practitioner's psyche. The sleepless nights, work-filled weekends, absence of vacations, strain placed on families and friends experienced by the clinical pharmacist today—where do these expectations of superhuman output come from? Actually, from the person peering right back at us in the mirror: ourselves.

Is this a view that I've personally always held? Not at all. I once embraced this work-centric mind-set with reckless ambition. It was nothing for me to work a 14-hour day and then go home with a stack of continued work items. I volunteered for every committee, task force, and research project available at my institution. My manager was constantly reminding me that I was no longer a resident and that I couldn't keep going at this pace for risk of burnout. This advice was taken by me from its original intent and used to further fuel my already zealous work-life obsession. This behavior continued for several years until I noticed something happening that I didn't want to admit; I couldn't do everything anymore. Talk about a humbling epiphany—but more on that later.

Not only are we responsible for these overzealous expectations placed on ourselves, but we also exhibit this behavior to the pharmacy students and residents we are mentoring. Our actions speak volumes to these futures of our profession, which should make us wonder—what are we really imparting to them? Sure, we teach skills in critical thinking, public presentation, data analysis, and provision of the best patient care possible. The traditional tools used to teach students are journal clubs, patient presentations, and drug utilization evaluations, among many others; all are effective options for student and resident learning. The problem is that, somewhere along the way, we neglect to teach these eager learners how to realistically use these tools to be productive versus busy and embarking on what I like to call the *Busy Cycle*.

The Busy Cycle is a concept that almost everyone in health care has seen in either themselves or a colleague. The Busy Cycle begins to spin as a person begins obsessing over the tasks to be done, but starts losing focus on the intent behind the tasks. Soon, those caught up in it are working at a frantic pace to keep their heads above water while losing touch with the basic concepts of patient care, which is the entire basis for our jobs. During my stint on the Busy Cycle, I would catch more and more of my own mistakes because I was so focused on what else I had to accomplish. Thankfully, none of these instances resulted in patient harm. One such occurrence happened early in my career when I was still fresh out of residency. I was working on a code blue course development, toiling through an MUE, and trying to perform my normal patient care duties. Soon, I was getting calls from nurses that medications were taking much longer than usual to be verified and delivered to the patient locations. It hit me like a ton of bricks that my focus had shifted from patient care to items on a to-do list. How did I jump on the Busy Cycle?

Perhaps many practicing pharmacists think mistakenly productivity and busyness are the same thing. To contribute to patient care, clinicians believe they must be continuously juggling precepting students, residents, research, pharmacoeconomic review, and various types of committee work, all while trying to provide safe pharmacotherapy to patients. In reality, the busier many practitioners are, the less productive they become because they never really complete anything meaningful. The infamous to-do list is full of items that never get crossed off because other tasks get added constantly. So why don't we teach our students and residents how to be productive instead of busy?

Truthfully, the reason most practicing clinicians neglect to teach workload management is that we don't have a good idea of how to do it ourselves—hence, the trickle-down of the Busy Cycle from mentor to preceptor to resident to student. Each level in the learning tree hierarchy feels perceived pressure to work harder and prove to their supervisor that they are achieving excellence. The reality is, each person who partakes in this frantic-paced workplace is driven by the perceived fear that someone will think he or she is not working up to certain standards. The residents and students who watch this process are brainwashed into believing that this is the only way to have a successful career. Taking home stacks of articles and journals to read during one's personal time should be something of one's choosing, not an expectation. Some preceptors will say that the workaholic lifestyle is a choice and that they are not forcing the student to follow their lead. This sounds good until the student gets an evaluation with comments such as "not working to full potential" or "lack of desire or motivation." This criticism is quite often carried with students as they become new practitioners, and then they adopt this obsessive work style with nothing driving them but fear of future critique. So how do we break the Busy Cycle? Should we break the Busy Cycle?

Both of these are very controversial and debatable questions, with associated benefits and consequences. I recently spoke with a physician colleague who is well known and highly respected, not only in the community but also as a pediatric health care political adviser, who told me a story about a grandiose physician who built a practice that was massive. The patients lined up for months to get an appointment at this prestigious practice, and the entire local medical community strived to emulate this model. Everyone talked about this great physician and his accomplishments all the time. When he finally retired from the empire he created, it took less than 2 months for people to completely forget about him and continue taking care of patients the way they always had. Not to mention that this once-iconic figure in the health care world had sacrificed two marriages and all of his children's youth activities to this practice that now continued flawlessly without him. This poor physician had been so obsessed with building and creating that he had never been able to break the Busy Cycle. Yet patient care was in existence before we joined the health care world, and it will continue after we exit it, no matter how much we feel that we are irreplaceable.

Another component of the Busy Cycle is the continuous pressure to expand pharmacy services into every aspect of patient care. Although this is a valid need given the amount of patient safety and improved outcomes seen with the addition of pharmacy services, pharmacy has a very precarious role in the health care team. Pharmacists are one of the most expensive components of the institutional budget because of the burden of medication procurement, yet the literature repeatedly shows that they save resources by their respective patient care services. Pharmacy workplace environments under a financial burden to cut all non-essential spending are increasing the workload on the staff without increasing the staff numbers to compensate. Increased workload furthers job stress, home stress, and interdepartmental stress. New requirements for better pharmaceutical practices, increasing drug shortages, decreasing third-party reimbursement, and research into individualized medication therapy all contribute to larger roles of pharmacists in the medical care of patients. Yet these requirements lead to shorter deadlines and increased levels of stress. So how do we keep from jumping on the Busy Cycle with reckless abandonment?

The first and most obvious step is to examine our own work styles and decide what we are actually accomplishing. Are we doing work that will positively affect patient care, or are we buried in the realm of busy work? Do we spend the necessary time evaluating the impact of our interventions and projects, or do we frantically finish one task only to dive right into the next? Spending countless hours on a presentation that contains merely reformatted information is not productive time. If we, as practitioners, were to honestly and objectively evaluate our working time on two critical points—busy work and impactful work—I'm afraid that many of us might find the majority of our efforts landing in the former realm.

Please do not interpret this notion of overworking as an excuse to plod through the day at a snail's pace. Rather, give yourself, and those you are responsible for, a realistic and accomplishable amount of work, and prioritize the items that will affect patient care. I have taken the approach that no matter how much work I try to cram into a day, there will always be some left over for tomorrow. Using the SMART goal strategy for daily activities has completely refocused my job and its rationale. *Specifying* the goals for the day and making them *measurable* helps me focus on the essential daily tasks. Assessing the *achievability* and *realistic* probability of the daily objectives eliminates the items that are too lofty and ambitious. Finally, the *timeliness* of each item forces me to prioritize the most time-sensitive items that must be completed first. By making myself critically sort and organize each daily activity into these five categories, I find that I'm able to complete the appropriate amount of work in the appropriate amount of time.

To illustrate this strategy, let me use a personal example from the not-too-distant past. I had a CE article to write, a MUE manuscript submission deadline looming, two IRB-approved studies needing data analysis, employee evaluations, and the normal daily duties of a pharmacy manager. I sorted the tasks by when they were due, allowing me to focus on the most time-sensitive items. The employee evaluations were due in 3 weeks, which would normally move them to the top of the list. However, the manuscript and CE submission would need to be reviewed and returned by the journal editors, which meant they should be done first. My duties of meetings, committee work, and scheduling have to be done daily, which puts them in the race for top completion priority. Data analysis takes a long time and requires complete focus, so it made perfect sense that this should be *numero uno*. Hence the question: how could I organize this monstrous list when all items were a top priority? By looking objectively at the list and removing my own personal bias, I could see that not all of the tasks were time-sensitive and that they could be prioritized with the SMART method. The data analysis tasks were still an early part of the study process and were therefore not close to being done. The CE article date for publication was not yet set, so a deadline for submission could not be generated. The employee evaluations needed peer evaluation comments in addition to self-evaluation, so they required others' help to complete. The MUE manuscript had a defined submission deadline and was finished, save for a few formatting issues. The daily tasks would be there regardless of all other pressing needs. In less than 5 minutes, I determined that I needed to focus my energy on completing my daily tasks, the MUE submission, the employee evaluations, the CE article, and then the data analysis. By looking at the *specifics* of each task, I found the *achievability* and *reality* of task completion much easier to determine. Accurately measuring the *timeliness* of each task and the time until the deadline is also critical to proper prioritization.

The last step is to explain and demonstrate to younger practitioners how to meet deadlines and expectations, guiding and enabling them to succeed. Yet if deadlines and expectations are not realistic and achievable by a clinician, they are just another item on an infinitely expanding to-do list. Expecting future pharmacy professionals to learn and perform at a high level without modeling for them how to be productive versus busy is simply continuing the vicious Busy Cycle.

One of the great strategies in combating the Busy Cycle is open communication between professional colleagues. As previously stated, it is incredibly easy to compare your work output with that of a colleague and to feel pressured to keep up with peers. I have often witnessed that this is a misinterpretation of colleagues and that a quick conversation about current projects can highlight the true state of the workload. Additionally, veteran practitioners should be willing to discuss with new practitioners the need to focus on quality output versus quantity of busy work. By creating a sense of teamwork and a professional support structure, the Busy Cycle is less likely to spin out of control.

It is quite clear, by examining the past 25 years' growth in pharmacy services outside traditional dispensing roles, that our profession has come an extraordinarily long way. Should this growth continue on its trajectory, there is no way to accurately project where pharmacy will be in 2036. However, along with this growth and demand for pharmacy services, there will surely be an increase in workload output, which will further complicate the balance of busyness and productivity. It is critical that we begin now to reflect on our own practices, examining the type of professional behavior we exude. Are we the clinicians who produce quality patient care while understanding our own limits? Or are we the overworked, stressed-out, and task-obsessed clinicians who focus on the to-do list and miss the concept of quality patient care? Finally, how can we mold the future professionals of pharmacy to provide the level of patient care that we all know is critical if we don't first break the Busy Cycle? My opinion is that, until we fix ourselves, we cannot begin to teach our students and residents—the futures of our profession—these important life skills.

There Are No Pharmacists on *Star Trek*

Donald Zabriskie, BPharm, MBA, RPh
Clinician/Educator

There are no pharmacists on *Star Trek*.
Wait a minute! Hear me out.

There have been medical technicians, salesmen, farmers, chefs, many bartenders, and, as you likely know (but won't admit that you know it), a good number of physicians. Dr. McCoy, Dr. Crusher, Dr. Bashir, the holographic doctor, and Dr. Phlox. And nurses? I could list those as well, starting with Nurse Christine Chapel (she of the golden blonde beehive hairdo!). But no pharmacists, druggists, chemists, or apothecaries.

In all 704 episodes of the television show and in the 11 movies, you never once saw a pharmacist. Certainly not on the *Enterprise* and never even during the planet-side adventures of the crew.

The reality check is that it was just a television show and a lucrative franchise property for the studios. But given the many professions that did show up in all of those hours, why didn't one single scriptwriter think of throwing in a pharmacist? They were writing in an era when a pharmacist was consistently the most trusted professional around in the United States. What happened?

The pharmacist in the twenty-fourth century simply doesn't exist!

If we distill down the perceived skills of the pharmacist and of the clinical pharmacist, in particular, we can easily supplant the person with the technology that will be available in the twenty-fourth century. Our drugs will be created using replicator technology, and we'll have a voice-responsive computer everywhere we go to get information about the drug.

But why should you or I worry? This is way, way, way in the fictional future. Except the future is pretty much here today.

Drug preparation doesn't really exist much in the twenty-first century. Many pharmacists in practice today would be challenged to prepare an ointment or even a capsule version of a medication. Even in a modern hospital, literally every preparation is prepackaged, premixed, or otherwise within one step of its final form, whether it's an intravenous piggyback medication or a peritoneal dialysis solution.

Drug distribution? We've already moved to automated drug distribution systems by the twenty-first century, let alone the twenty-fourth century. Connect a drug-filled ATM with prescriber order entry and intelligent logic programs, and pharmacists themselves are extraneous to drug distribution throughout the nation's hospitals. And in community practice, we're already seeing similar dispensing systems, albeit in the early stages of development.

And drug information? I'm not as technically savvy as many of you, but I am carrying around a huge amount of drug information in my mobile device—more than existed in a pharmacology reference from the mid-1980s. And that would be a great resource for a pharmacist's use until you remembered that anyone like a salesman, chef, or even a bartender with the appropriate subscription and online access through a smart device has the same information at his fingertips. The mystery of the drug information service with its special journal subscriptions and access to a variety of esoteric databases has evaporated as the Internet, and access to it, has exploded across the entire globe.

This ability to access drug information resources encompasses patients as well. You have to know that I am a little more "on my toes" with a patient when I look across the room and see his personal laptop up and running, hooked into the hospital's wireless system, while he asks me questions about his drug therapy.

We are victims of our own predilection for intellectual perfection rather than understanding our true worth in yesterday's, today's, and the future's health care environment.

This pursuit of intellectual capital resulted in the move to an entry-level degree consisting of 6 years (or longer) of study and rotations. Then, segments of the organized profession decided that academia was incapable of producing a competent practitioner, giving us the latest move to tack on at least 1 year of residency to really prepare the pharmacist to practice. We have begun to create a profession of elites right at a time when elite services will not survive the economic environment of the 2020s.

We have yielded our position as the drug expert by the mere fact that there are not as many of us as there are nurses. The nation's hospitals, recognizing the need for that human touch together with up-to-date drug information, have nurses fulfilling the pharmacist's primary role. Hospitals do acknowledge the expertise of the pharmacist. But the pressures to improve HCAHPS scores won't be relieved by the paltry number of highly compensated (compared with nurses) pharmacists available to meet with patients about new drugs. This has been and will continue to be another burden for the already overburdened staff nurse.

The pharmacist cannot be content to have the role of patron saint of drug information who guides the nurse to the correct resources. Patients will not be content with the necessarily perfunctory attention given to drug information that the nurse can deliver.

Pharmacists need to reestablish their traditional connection to the patient and maintain it for the foreseeable future.

Patients want to be counseled. They want to talk with the pharmacist. What they have needed, need, and will need is a health care professional who looks them in the eye and tells them what a drug is called, what it will treat, the bad things that could happen (well, tactfully and in context), and then opens up to any question about drug therapy. An Internet resource or an automated drug distribution system can't softly touch the hand of the 83-year-old who is new to warfarin therapy or firmly grip the hand in a heartfelt handshake of the 52-year-old pneumonia patient who just wants to know that he has the right drugs and that someone is watching over his drug therapy.

When people ask me how I got started in pharmacy, I try to put a bit of a self-deprecating spin on the tale. It was the latter part of the 1960s when my mother made me take a job helping in an old-style independent community pharmacy. You know the kind. Driving the Dodge Dart to deliver prescriptions. Cleaning the store. Loading the soft drink machine. Brown paper wrapping of feminine hygiene products. One pharmacist drove a black T-Bird, and both of the owners lived way out in the suburbs in beautiful homes. And all they had to do was be able to count 5, 10, 15, 20, and so on. What a life! Because you never even had to tell the patient what they were taking or why they were taking it. My punch line is that here I was anticipating a blissful life of nice cars, nice homes, and no need for patient involvement, and then what comes along today? Patients who want to know all about their drugs. Patients who need to know all about their drugs. Patients with questions. What happened to my planned simple life?

But in reality, I saw and felt the personal connection that the two old-school pharmacists had with patients. Patients looked up to these pharmacists. They were the health professional you confided in, sought advice from, and truly listened to. I kid about a legacy that includes fast cars and nice homes, but I have nothing but the utmost reverence for the way I was brought up in the profession. I've never questioned whether or not a pharmacist has a role in health care. I am a caregiver, and I hope that this will be true for pharmacists for years to come.

Periodically, the pharmacy profession loses its way. And on a regular basis, the profession tries to find its way back to the one true path. From the corner druggist dispensing sage advice and nostrums to the concept of pharmaceutical care to the current revelation that a new pharmacy practice model is needed: all had the same message.

Patients need and want the personal intervention of a pharmacist. The profession needs the tenets of the current pharmacy practice model initiative and, this time, needs to stick to them. Because failure to follow this path will hasten the inexorable march to the pharmacist-free future you see on *Star Trek*.

If this time we stick to the plan and start delivering the type of health care we are so good at, maybe in the newly conceived *Star Trek* franchise, we'll have a chance to hear the dialog:

Kirk· "Spock, Bones! We need someone in the Eridani 49 orbiting medical facility that has medical knowledge, administrative skills, and can show empathy for a race of reptilian quadrupeds."

McCoy: "Damn it, Jim! I'm a doctor, not a pharmacist!"

Spock: "Fascinating, Doctor. A logical choice for a change."

Recognizing Limitations

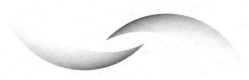

The fundament upon which all our knowledge and learning rests is the inexplicable.

Arthur Schopenhauer

The heart has its reasons, which reason does not know.

Blaise Pascal

Sometimes a scream is better than a thesis.

Ralph Waldo Emerson

An Encounter in Patient Care

Joel Henneberry, Pharm.D. Candidate 2012
Student

I am finding that it actually takes work to keep an open mind. It isn't something easily grasped, as harsh experiences drown the vitality of a once youthful and hopeful self. However difficult, I find it necessary. Without an open mind, you see a person only as a member of a group; you label him or her each according to things that remind you of other persons. From this, you gain the power of intuition, but you lose the power of innocence, and the patient is the one who loses when your intuition grinds out another mistaken perception, another wrong label. An open mind to me means seeing people for everything they are worth as human beings, seeing every person as an individual, deserving of whatever help can be given. I learned something about keeping an open mind in an encounter I observed in the field. We don't talk about this sort of thing in school.

The very first patient I saw when rounding with the medical team changed my paradigm of health care. He was lying under thin sheets and wearing thick black-rimmed glasses. His hospital gown hung loosely off his bony white shoulders, and his skin was speckled with brown age spots. He was mostly bald, with some thin hair darkened by dried sweat near his temples. I'll call him "Marty" for privacy's sake. He reached over for his wooden cane and leaned it closer to the bed.

Since this was a teaching hospital, there was a whole crowd of us waddling in, wearing white coats; we were a string of sheep following our gray-haired shepherd—the attending physician. We crowded around Marty's bed, our bodies forming a temporary sound barrier, muting the busy hospital noise from outside in the hall. Marty smiled as we all introduced ourselves: medical intern, residents, student pharmacists, and all. He responded kindly to the attending physician, calling him Doc as they talked between open mouth breaths and listening to the heart and lungs.

Under cordial overtones, it became apparent that Doc and Marty could not have been on further spectrums of the idea of health care.

"How are you doing?" asked the doctor.

"Not great, Doc. I can't sleep here at night; there is too much noise in the hallway," he said. "I want to go home."

The doctor paused to sit on the edge of the bed.

"Marty," the doctor said. "I'm not comfortable letting you go yet."

"I have to go home, Doc. I can't eat the food here. It hurts my stomach."

The attending physician smiled, took off his glasses, and rubbed his eyes. "Marty," he said. "You have to understand, it's because of your condition that I can't let you go. I need some more time to monitor your heart. I don't think it has fully recovered yet."

Marty continued in his deliberate efforts. "I have the best nurse in the world at home."

The doctor gestured to object, but Marty continued. "My wife. She is the best nurse in the world."

The physician gave it one last shot, trying to protect the patient from all harm—perhaps even from himself. "Marty, I need you to understand, if you leave right now, without all of us here, and the medicine and the machines to help you," he paused for effect, "you could die in the next few hours, or the next few days."

It was like Marty knew only one song. "We have been married 41 years, Doc. She's the best nurse in the world."

The doctor looked up at all of us, scanning our faces to read our thoughts. We looked around at each other, surprised at the drama playing out this early in the morning. I could see in the doc's watering eyes and faint smile that Marty had struck deep emotions in this old physician. After a few more moments of reflection, the doctor chose his words legally.

"Marty, I need you to understand something. If I let you go now, it is against my best judgment as a physician. You have to understand that I will put in the report that you will be leaving AMA, against medical advice. Would you consider staying just one night more?"

"She's a great cook, too."

We all laughed with Marty this time. "OK, Marty," said the gray-haired physician as he patted Marty's frail leg and replaced his own glasses.

"Goodbye, Doc." Marty said quietly. "Thank you."

Marty smiled again at all of us as we shuffled out of his room. As I shut the door, he gave me one last smile, put his hands behind his head, and rested back on his pillow. I bet I know who he was thinking about.

And so it was that a 15-minute experience with a patient changed my perspective on health care. I could no longer think of patients as we had in school, on paper, fitting neatly into the therapy regimens we set, also on paper. Patients, I realized, are each their own story. They come to us at different chapters. Some are in an introductory battle with random illness, wandering shell-shocked into our hospital beds, jolted from daily routine by an ambush against which none could have prepared. Others are at a low point, lost among the consequences of poor life choices, desperately grasping our extended hands. Some are at a climax, starting down a new path toward a healthier lifestyle, one choice at a time. Some, like Marty, are coming to us at sunset. We bring the tools we know to the table, while he brings his life. We hunt the sickness like predators, but it is the patient who can save us from ourselves, who can release us from our duty. In the end, the very end, the body fails. Marty chose to spend an hour longer with his wife than to stay with us and fight it out in the unpleasant battle zones of health care. So we must temper our goals for each patient's care, to meet their true needs, whether we understand them or not. To me, this is the essence of keeping an open mind, so that I can take each patient as an independent and important human being, not bound by my preconceived notions of what health care might mean to them.

Faith?

Stephen W. Janning, Pharm.D.
Clinician

Hardly a day passes without another report of a suicide bomber wreaking death and destruction somewhere in the Middle East. The reasons the bomber chooses this path are undoubtedly complex, but a common theme is self-sacrifice. In essence, they "die for their faith." The reaction to the news of these faraway tragedies depends in part on one's point of view regarding the professed faith of the person sacrificing him/herself. In this example, what represents a brave and admirable act to some (martyrdom) is considered an abhorrent expression of misguided faith to most others (murder). However, outside these extremes, which perhaps include politically motivated examples, dying for one's faith is a mysterious event that very few have actually witnessed.

More than 20 years ago, a woman was admitted to an inner-city hospital for the management of blunt abdominal trauma sustained during a motor vehicle crash. I was the clinical pharmacist working with the trauma surgery team. During the initial evaluation, it was established that she was a Jehovah's Witness and would require blood product transfusions to survive the necessary surgery. A serious conflict of interest because that religion forbids blood transfusions.

The team was skeptical, in the way that many intensive care clinicians inure themselves to the cold realities of their work. No problem. We'd seen this scenario many times before. The only questions to resolve were, which category of "Jehovah's Witness Lite" would she fall into and when. In our experience, they always eventually ended up accepting a transfusion when their life was on the line. Some would hold out and not allow anything containing erythrocytes. Others would literally beg for any transfusion once the consequences of not doing so were made clear. But the Witnesses always folded in the end.

Not this time.

oxygen delivery = (oxygen-carrying capacity × cardiac output)
cardiac output = (stroke volume × heart rate)

Those simple physiology relationships had never before seemed quite so cruel. The patient's heart rate began to climb. There simply wasn't enough oxygen being delivered because of her significant intra-abdominal bleeding. Soon, her heart would lose the battle and simply infarct itself in spite of maximized crystalloid intravascular volume repletion. The team spoke with the patient, who was quite lucid throughout. She steadfastly refused any and all transfusions. Her family, staying by her side in the surgical intensive care unit, concurred. They were almost eerily calm about the situation, believing that their God would either save her or take her to a better place when it was over.

The usual suspects were called in: social worker, psychiatrist, pastoral care. The patient remained staunchly committed to her decision, and the consultants confirmed that she was quite competent to do so. The team watched in apprehension, fearing the inevitable outcome much more than the patient. We kept returning to her bedside, wanting to be ready to "save her" when she changed her mind. Eventually, most of us just stayed put, transfixed by what we were seeing. She died before our eyes in a completely serene state, believing to the very end that she had already been saved by staying true to the path her faith demanded.

That was the single most courageous act I have ever personally witnessed. I still think about it from time to time. I still can't say for sure that I fully comprehend or completely agree with her decision. But I know that I deeply respect it. Perhaps what makes it so difficult to understand is that it reflects a depth of faith that many profess but that comparatively few truly possess and fewer still have the conviction or courage to express in such absolute terms. The team's faith was in Western medicine and its power to heal and "save," which by comparison seems rather shallow, in a strictly philosophical sense. Maybe that's why we were the ones who were afraid.

We have an obligation to make available and thoroughly explain the risks and benefits of all treatment options to our patients. This includes the option of "doing nothing." The ultimate decision remains with the patient, even if we don't agree with it, even if we don't understand it. Even if it means death. That was a powerful lesson for a young practitioner just 2 years out of residency training.

I have no doubt that many, perhaps most, suicide bombers are mentally ill individuals, many of whom are victimized by political extremists to conduct heinous acts in the name of their God. I do not at all believe that any true religion, as I understand the concept, advocates retribution against anyone by means of random mass murder. But I absolutely believe that, for a few, there exists a depth of faith that is literally worth dying for. I've seen it.

Mr. Green's Blue Pills

J. Christopher Lynch, Pharm.D.
Clinician

Quitting time comes early in New Orleans on the last Friday afternoon of Carnival, leaving me the only staff member in the Charity Hospital Diabetes Clinic at 4:30. I sat near an open window as I finished reviewing the last refill requests of the week, hoping in vain for a trickle of fresh air to overcome the blast of heat from the gurgling iron radiators. From Tulane Avenue eight stories below came the happy, slightly hysterical sounds of an early Mardi Gras season evening. Taxis packed with tourists crawled past en route to the Quarter, their mufflers rumbling and the passengers' Caligulan fantasies finding expression in yips of glee and guttural rebel yells.

I called in my last refill, commiserating with the retail pharmacist about the constant stream of drunken frat boys she'd faced all day; filed the charts away on the rack; and made the last rounds, flipping off light switches and closing the open windows. With my hand on the final switch, I heard someone rapping on the outer door, long since locked. It wasn't a knocking, but a rapping, as if someone was tentatively testing out a new battering ram. I opened the door and found Mr Green, an old—very old—patient of mine, his chin held high and his hardwood cane cocked for another rap.

Even at 93 years old and standing 5 feet flat, Mr. Green cut quite a figure. He dressed each day as if he might be called upon to run for alderman or to deliver the closing arguments in a murder trial. Shoes shined, nails buffed, creases razor sharp. If he'd had any hair, I'm sure it would've been perfect. As it was, his head reminded me of a particularly exotic egg—speckled, brown, and flawlessly oiled. Mr. Green was one of those very rare men who didn't seem ridiculous in an ascot. If you sought someone to play him in a movie shot in 1978, you could have done no better than to cast Scatman Crothers. *Love Boat* Scatman, not *The Shining*.

He had been a patient of the clinic for years, and I knew him well. He was a part-time minister, part-time bookie, and full-time flirt who missed appointments with abandon and expected to be seen by any specialist he could name immediately upon his unscheduled arrival. He would occasionally appear without medical request, merely to loaf around the waiting room and talk about his plans to relocate to southern Florida. "I'm gonna get me a high-rise condo and a low-rent woman," he would say. Mr. Green was a rascal, and we loved him.

"Good afternoon, Doc," he said, sweeping past me. "I've come for some hard-on pills."

Now, this was in the early days of Viagra, when it was still a topic bandied about on local newscasts and often served as the punch line of weak late-night monologues. But it was also back in the day when prescribers were justifiably nervous of the potential cardiovascular implications of allowing a man who had been sedentary for decades to obtain the erection of a 17-year-old boy. So, cardiac stress testing was required before the magic blue pills were dispensed. Absolutely mandatory. No exceptions.

While Mr. Green was an inveterate and tireless pitcher of woo, and no woman from the freshest nursing student to the most grizzled unit secretary was safe from his tireless advances, I had always assumed that his days of active sexuality had faded away sometime during the Reagan administration. To me, at age 30 or so, the idea of Mr. Green asking for help obtaining a quality erection was as absurd as a toddler enquiring about the purchase of a handgun. It just wasn't something I would ever expect him to need or, quite frankly, anything I would want to think about his using. But there he was.

I pulled his chart and found what I expected; Mr. Green had been prescribed Viagra and issued paperwork for a cardiac stress test, but he had never appeared at the lab. No stress test, no more Viagra. When I relayed the bad news, Mr. Green's amiable expression darkened immediately.

"I'm not leaving here without them, Doc. I have a hot date tonight, and I need those pills. If you want to make the Krewe d'Etat parade, I suggest you hustle."

I found myself unsure what to do. It wasn't a problem legally, as I had standing orders that covered such things and, after many years, the full trust of my medical director and attending physicians. And here he was, apparently as hale and hearty as anyone could wish, with a very reasonable request. Reasonable in his mind at least. If he had been 20 years younger and my mind could have processed the idea of him having sex, perhaps it would've been easier to say yes. But my own biases, my deep-seated reluctance to accept the sexuality of this man nearing his century mark, somehow set my brain on tilt.

"You have a date?" was all I could find to say.

"I do, and she isn't a woman to be kept waiting."

Fogbound, I opened the sample closet. There they were, row upon row of little blue boxes, each containing three of the little blue pills that had so caught the communal imagination. I took one down and signed it out.

"How about two boxes, Doc? It's a long weekend."

"No, sir. One box is all. It has three pills. That will be plenty for the weekend." I pressed the box into his hand and locked his eyes with mine. "And I want you here Wednesday morning for your stress test. No exceptions."

"OK, Doc," he said, his face again alive with his charming smile. "Wednesday morning. I promise."

He left the clinic with me, pausing for a moment as I locked the door. "I can't tell you what this means to me, Doc. I need this more than anything right now."

Still, I doubted the existence of his date. But we turned the corner to the elevators, and there she was. Easily 80, she stood clutching her purse to her chest, eyes shining, looking as frail and angular as old origami.

"Did you get 'em?" she asked.

"The Doc here set us up," he said, tapping the box against his palm.

"Oh, bless you, baby," she said, beaming up at me.

As we rode down in the creaking chrome elevator I noticed her inching closer and closer to him until their hips were gently touching. Their hands entwined, fingers rubbing with a sound like fine-grit sandpaper. After we stepped off and separated on the ground floor, I saw her give his hand a big squeeze and saw him pat her gently on the behind with the hand that held his cane.

Mr. Green never did come back for that cardiac stress test. In fact, I never saw the old rascal again. Sometimes, I worry that I did a horribly wrong thing. But most of the time, I hope that he had one last great Mardi Gras weekend before he finally moved south to Florida.

Chicago

Lori Wilken, Pharm.D., BS
Clinician

I work in Chicago. Not in the tourist section or the North Shore. My job is to help people stop smoking. I have my own clinic that doctors from every type of specialty refer their patients to for treatment. This has been my job for the past 15 years. I have never smoked a day in my life. It doesn't matter.

Last week was a busy week in clinic. The weather was warming up a bit, and Easter was almost here. New hope. I see patients in an exam room in a clinic. Individual appointments. A box of generic, scratchy, paper-thin tissues are close by before I call a patient into the room. I always have a smile on my face.

My first patient is not new to me. She has been in clinic before. She smokes ½ pack of Newports a day. She has an 8-year-old son who wants her to quit smoking. She wants to quit smoking. She sees a psychiatrist every week because she has post-traumatic stress disorder. Her ex-husband would smash her head against a wall, and now she has headaches and seizures and pain. She just wants to go back to school and get her master's degree and work again. She wants to be a good role model for her son. "Why is it so hard to quit smoking?"

My second patient comes in and wants to kill her mother. She has interstitial lung disease, and she is 43 years old. A pack of smokes is gone in no time. "If my mother does not get out of my house by tomorrow, I swear I will kill her!" Her mother was the one who watched her be molested as a child by each new boyfriend that came to stay at the house. Her mother was the one who was supposed to protect her. "I want to live."

My third patient comes in, and he is a carpenter. He just got laid off work. He quit smoking in the past for 6 months using the patches. He is a proud father of three children and happily married. He relapsed when his oldest son came back from fighting in Afghanistan. His son, who had *Neisseria meningitidis*, had not been home even 1 month when he died. He had tears in his eyes as he described his son's children and the arguments with the daughter-in-law over the funeral arrangements. "I need to quit."

The last patient of the day had third-degree burns all over her body. The clinical notes say that a man threw gasoline all over her and her son and then lit a match. That was not what was hurting her today. Her husband of 23 years threw her and their young daughter out of their home. Homeless. "I can quit smoking."

I once had a sociology professor in college who said people with psychiatric illnesses were not really the ill people. The people that can watch all of the madness in the world and still have a smile on their faces were really the sick people. Now I understand. Doctors, priests, social workers, and now *pharmacists* are in positions where they are asked to really listen to each person. It is painful and difficult to hear the truth, so we become numb. This numbness is not intentional or vicious; it is a means of survival. My smile has to be indifferent. Should I stop smiling? I believe the patients need some form of hope. Should I change jobs? I think this is part of the "illness." I really enjoy my work. I empathize with the patients "painfully" to the point of tears when no one is around. I believe the patients have empathy for me, too. So much so that they may not return to clinic if they believe that I cannot handle "their truth." Can anything be done? For the patients, they need to be heard. For me, the pharmacist, it is a maturing process. It is accepting reality.

Humanizing the Profession

Educating the mind without educating the heart is no education at all.

Aristotle

The greatest mistake in the treatment of diseases is that there are physicians for the body and physicians for the soul, although the two cannot be separated.

Plato

One of the most valuable things we can do to heal one another is listen to each others' stories.

Rebecca Falls

Empathy: Putting Students Back in Touch with Their Right Brains

Chad A. Knoderer, Pharm.D.
Educator

Laurie L. Pylitt, M.H.P.E., PA-C
Educator

Is medicine or, better yet, patient care, an art or a science? It's a delicate balance of both. When combined, science, data, facts, and outcomes balanced with perspective, relationships, sympathy, and empathy lead to good medicine and good patient care. Ask most pharmacy students why they chose the field of pharmacy, and they will tell you that they are good at math and science and that they are, overall, conscientious students—that they are good manipulators of information. Probe deeper, and students will also report that they chose pharmacy as a career because they wanted to help people. They chose pharmacy because it would allow them to balance science, data, facts, and outcomes with perspective, relationships, sympathy, and empathy.

From the time most pharmacy students arrive at their respective universities (and probably even before) until they leave, they are focused on closely manipulating information associated with left-brain functions. A perusal of the CAPE[1] document reinforces that the preponderance of outcomes relies on the acquisition, manipulation, and analysis of pharmacy and drug-related information. Thus, it is logical that pharmacy students spend most of their time, especially in the early years of their education, acquiring information.

Daniel Pink[2] and others argue that this real-world knowledge is necessary but no longer sufficient to be successful in one's work. The contributions of the right brain—synthesis, emotional expression, context, and the big picture—also play a major role in building successful careers and productive societies. The CAPE outcomes[1] delineate the need to communicate with patients, considering the ethical, social, and economic context. In most pharmacy programs, the curriculum structure defers to the APPE experiences in students' final years of training to refine the "art" of pharmacy represented by the CAPE communication outcome. This curricular structure creates a great divide for students as they transition from their science (left brain) years in the early part of their education to the final, high-stakes APPE experiences, during which (right brain) interactions with patients and others are key to their success.

Today's pharmacy curriculum allows little time for pharmacy educators to integrate right-brain perspectives as they deliver lectures, share clinical experiences, or lead case discussions. However, it is a remarkably short journey from the time students enter college until they are faced with patients, families, and caregivers in various stages of health, illness, and, at times, death. So, in addition to acquiring clinical knowledge and developing problem-solving abilities, students need to learn how to appreciate perspective, develop relationships, and exhibit compassion to grasp the big picture of patient care. Encouraging students to step out of the box and out of their comfort zones and to get in touch with their right-brain reasons for choosing to become pharmacists is challenging. It is important for educators to create opportunities in which students can appreciate that patients (even if they are only paper cases discussed in class) are people with feelings and emotions.

At Butler University, we recently challenged our students with an assignment focused on getting in touch with their right brains. When we introduced the assignment, we used a quotation to help put the importance of right-brain functions in proper perspective:

Nobody cares how much you know, until they know how much you care.

—Theodore Roosevelt

The assignment tasked students in their third professional year (about 6 weeks before APPEs) with finding something meaningful to help them connect a disease state or therapeutic intervention to the "human" side of patients when practicing as a pharmacist. Their chosen item could have been anything, such as a painting, video, book, movie, piece of art, patient-written letter, blog created for patients/ families with a specific disease, or personal reflection on an interaction with a patient. The selection was then posted to a group discussion page on a Web-based learning management system. Each student reflected on the reasons for choosing the item, their reaction when first encountering the item, and how the selection might change or affect their approach with patients as they began clinical rotations and ultimately their practice. Students were also asked to review and comment on contributions made by a small group (four or five) of their classmates. Finally, during the last week of classes, students presented their postings to the entire class in large-group format. The ultimate goal of the assignment was to expand the students' empathy and sympathy for others, encourage students to take the perspective of those who speak, have students view personal experiences and first-person stories as important ways of learning, and encourage students to embrace an ethic of caring. Upon completing the assignment, students participated in a SurveyMonkey evaluation of the exercise.

Our subsequent reflection on the assignment and student responses was enlightening and rewarding. Overwhelmingly, students felt that identifying and reflecting on an item connecting a disease state or intervention back to the patient or human side helped them see illness and disease from a perspective different from what had been taught in the classroom. Students' understanding of the patients' and caregivers' perspectives of disease was enhanced through the assignment. Students also felt a greater interest in using their roles as pharmacists to develop strategies to support the patient and caregiver.

The following statements summarize student perception of the assignment as collected from the anonymous online survey.

"The assignment was a good way to look at health care in a different perspective since the patient's well-being outside of the disease state is often put on the 'back burner' during class discussions."

"It is very difficult to teach empathy and emotions."

"The discussions in class are very clinical and impersonal to the patient, so it is encouraging to see what a big impact one can make by just taking a few extra seconds to sympathize with the patient or their family."

"I think that we all have the ability to be understanding and empathetic, and this assignment helps students see how they can be a positive influence on patients."

"Students don't get to do things like this in most classes, and it reinforced why we entered pharmacy school."

The timing of our assignment could not have been better to reinforce the "caring" aspect of patient care. However, an empathy assignment placed within the final semester before clinical rotations was bound to get a mixed reaction, and this exercise was no exception. A few students thought the assignment had no value in a pharmacy course, as evidenced by their insightful comments. One student stated: "I do not think this assignment was very worthwhile. I think that people either have compassion or they don't, and it is not something that we can learn." Another said: "While I feel like this assignment was very beneficial, doing a re-cap on the last day of class was kind of a depressing end to 5 long years of class."

Some may disagree about compassion as a learned trait. Compassion resides within all of us to some degree. What can be agreed on is that compassion or empathy or right-brain thinking plays a significant role in patient care, regardless of one's position as a pharmacist, prescriber, nurse, or student. As educators, we shouldn't wait for a single assignment at the end of 5 long years of didactic education or for the APPE experiences to help students stay connected with the right-brain reasons for their career choice. We must do what we have asked students to do: step out of the box and out of our comfort zones and find pedagogies throughout the didactic curriculum that will keep students connected with the right-brain reasons that led them to choose pharmacy as their career.

1. Center for the Advancement of Pharmaceutical Education Educational Outcomes 2004, American Association of Colleges of Pharmacy. Available at www.aacp.org/resources/education/Documents/CAPE2004.pdf. Accessed March 10, 2011.
2. Pink DH. A Whole New Mind: Why Right-Brainers Will Rule the Future. New York: Riverhead Books, 2006.

Sounds of Students

Judith L. Kristeller, Pharm.D., BCPS
Educator

As an educator, I facilitate the transition from student to practitioner throughout students' pharmacy education. This professionalism begins in year 1, but it becomes most apparent during the final experiential year of pharmacy school and is unique to each student. Reflective writing, especially during experiential learning, is one method to help students identify and assess their own personal and professional development. Without reflection, the professionalism of students becomes the tree that falls with nobody around to hear a sound.

Pharmacy educators need special tools to help students interpret and understand their professional maturation. Similar to optometrists, who need to use special vasodilators and lenses to see deep into our eyes, we need to look into our students to help them identify their emotional response to everyday professional issues. For example, after an excellent case presentation involving a critically ill patient with multiple sclerosis (MS), Lindsay reflected on what she had learned in the process as well as on her own dear friend with MS. In her reflection, she wrote,

> I spent quite a bit of time pouring over the information I had, only to come to the conclusion that there was nothing I could recommend to help my patient. To think of my friend getting to this point was a thought that soon followed. The whole situation not only made me feel inadequate in my knowledge concerning the disease and its treatment, but also a little hopeless. I was really trying to hold back these feelings when I was presenting.

As her mentor, I need to help Lindsay identify and not ignore her feelings so that her very normal response of feeling "inadequate" and "hopeless" is not confused with her own assessment of her ability as a pharmacist.

The topic of death is often overlooked, but it becomes inescapable during the pharmacy experience. We teach students about chronic progressive disease and ways to improve and prolong life. So is death the ultimate failure? If we deny students the opportunity to reflect on dying, we perpetuate the current health care model, in which dying is something discussed in the last few days of life because we would rather avoid the topic. Every physician, nurse, pharmacist, relative, and patient has their own view and their own plan. The patient with MS survived, but the experience helped Lindsay reflect on dying. A few weeks later, she wrote,

> When is it time to give up on someone? What if they have more fight in them? What if you are just prolonging the inevitable and ultimately causing waste or suffering? I don't know, but I'm sure these questions are something each practitioner has to deal with in their careers and answer for themselves.

Coming to terms with our own mortality is a natural aspect of personal and professional maturity. After reflection, we become more comfortable talking about these difficult issues with patients and colleagues. The reflective process helps students understand that they can maintain their professionalism, despite questioning some deeply personal issues.

I watch the transformation from nervous students to confident professionals. During this process, I need to help students find and balance their confidence, with their developing ability, and their clinical equipoise. Somewhere along this transition, the student takes over the reins of his or her education. One student wrote, "I recognized that there is always room for improvement, and that learning from your mistakes is more important than forgetting about them." Another wrote, "I've come to the realization that I am never going to know everything, but I can prepare for anything." We need to make sure we assess our students fairly, offer constructive suggestions, and give them time to reflect on the experience. As educators, we are part of the important process that builds a foundation to balance the personal and professional aspects of our lives, an interplay that is unique to each individual...and a "sound" that can only be heard by those who listen.

Accomplishing from Within: Defining Your Own Success in a Professional Environment

Maurice D. Alexander, Pharm.D.
Resident

Benyam Muluneh, Pharm.D.
Resident

"Residency training can be so busy at times that we rarely have time to truly reflect on what we want out of our career." Those are the words of a medical resident reflecting on what she thought to be the challenges of professional postgraduate training. She explained the value of removing oneself from the demands of his or her daily practice to reflect on what is most fulfilling. It was not long after this conversation that an article titled "The Expectation Conundrum: Reflections from a Residency Class" was published in the February 15, 2011, issue of the *American Journal of Health-System Pharmacy* by Fuhs and colleagues.[1] The article discusses the influence of expectations on professional achievement. It explores the importance of having those who train the next generation of pharmacy professionals ensure that their own expectations are in line with those of the trainee so that the successes of the emerging generation are not minimized. It was then that we realized that many professionals may fall prey to a tainted view of what it means to succeed.

So often, we as young professionals get lost in the expectations and goals of those who have come before us. Adding even more pressure for emerging practitioners to achieve is a professional climate that has never been more competitive. As more students seek postgraduate training in the form of a residency,

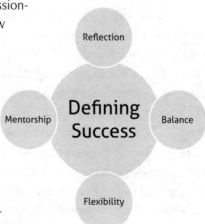

fellowship, etc., we are constantly looking for what will set us apart from our peers. In the effort to do great things, we often consult those whom we view as having already done great things, including highly regarded practitioners who are regionally/nationally respected, pharmacy leaders whose influence on the profession is unquestionable, and researchers whose work has shifted the way we practice pharmacy today. What we forget to do is consult ourselves.

Reflection
Defining individual paths for professional and personal success requires continuous reflection. Thorough reflection requires both historical and current perspectives to catapult oneself to a triumphant future. Reflecting is a very active process that requires specific steps to produce solid, measurable results. Often, this process is not encouraged or highlighted as an essential dimension of achieving success. We are often taught to broaden our networks, work on communication skills, and build key partnerships—in essence, focus on the "who we know." Although often neglected, "what we know," particularly about ourselves, is frequently the key to finding the prerequisite pieces to building our definition of success.

Reflection begins by attempting to retreat from others and work to correlate previous and current achievements to short- and long-term goals. These goals should be familiar and foundational but can be fluid and innovated over time. Doing this in regular time intervals allows a smooth process that results in continued development. Just as proper follow-up is crucial to ensuring that an intervention for a patient makes an enduring impact, careful meditation on our professional odyssey should be a pivotal piece of the professional development puzzle. Writing down our goals and aspirations and clearly tying these to the accomplishments that are fulfilling to ourselves, not others, allows an evaluation of the next steps. The next action item of reflection is to systematize and incorporate novel ideas to achieve our professional success. Retreating, writing, evaluating, and systematizing lead to the final step of reflection, which is evolving into our flourishing career to realize tangible, objective results birthed from our own reflective definitions of success.

Balance

Once we begin walking away from abstract expectations from external sources and start soaring toward our own defined reality of success, the ability to have a balanced life becomes essential. This balance should be valued as a vital piece to what has rendered one successful; it is not separate. What we do not advocate is eliminating mentors who hold us to high standards. They are valuable because they can help hold us accountable for the goals and successes we have outlined for ourselves. Therefore, the first skill is an ability to harmonize expected deeds with desired accomplishments. We are a society of emulators. Our understandings and measurements of success are made by using units set forth by our predecessors. Although it is not incorrect, this measurement unit of success is not always uniform. The globalization of certain units of measuring success often waters down the uniquely vibrant performances of many people. Individualization, reflection on critical values, and eventual ability to discover our own singular measurements of success are essential in our pursuit of genuine professional accomplishment.

Balance also suggests the ability to brew a series of lifetime achievements that blend both professional and personal dimensions. The professional and personal aspects of our lives often collaborate to create satisfaction and continued development. Incorrect perceptions that professional and personal successes are separate and mutually exclusive can be very distressing. Our definitions of success should always include the personal expectations we reflect on as well as our professional expectations. Creating the perfect balance of these two will establish the yin and yang concept: success in the careful unification of two superficially contrasting aspects of our lives.

Flexibility

Working toward achieving ultimate professional satisfaction necessitates the acceptance of fluidity in our goals and expectations. Having firm and foundational definitions and building on these over time is one formula for achieving self-defined professional success; however, working to modify these under various conditions (both positive opportunities and unfortunate circumstances) allows an extensive chiseling and reshaping of these expectations for eventual maturation.

Having a flexible perspective is advantageous when dealing with especially difficult situations. It is important not to forget that when we become resigned to the expectations of others, we cripple our ability to be flexible to our own evolving goals and circumstances. In addition, a person with a flexible attitude is one who is able to channel his or her aggression through patience. Although this novel concept of aggression through patience appears to be an oxymoron, it is essentially the ability to demonstrate an unwavering determination, even in trying situations, to arrive at the proposed expectation. In this context, an aggressive nature is not one of being belligerent and hostile, but rather, one of being dynamic and full of refreshing energy.

Mentorship

Although we have spent most of the article encouraging and challenging the reader to tap within to find his or her own definitions of success, a careful incorporation of the wisdom of senior practitioners is invaluable. We would like to stress that mentor selection should be deliberate and careful to ensure the mentee has a willing and able counselor to facilitate his or her idealistic expectations into realistic achievements. The mentor should never define the mentee's success. This requires that we responsibly appoint mentors whose expectations of our accomplishments are inspired by our own. Our experiences with our mentors are such that the mentors are very much external. Nevertheless, they are instrumental in conducting the concert rather than composing it.

Conclusion

Success is a personal fulfillment that only we, as individuals, can define for ourselves. As we read the expectation conundrum article alluded to above, the message that radiated was that falling victim to the expectations of others often induces a feeling of inadequacy, unworthiness, and inferiority. Reflecting on this, we could not help but apply the famous quote of Eleanor Roosevelt, "no one can make you feel inferior without your permission." If we consult ourselves first and define internally what it is that will declare us successful in our professional careers and in our personal lives, then the only way to fail is by failing ourselves, not others. This requires that we rid ourselves of the external influences and tap into what moves us internally as individuals. We happen to have a religious conviction that governs not only our personal lives, but also our professional goals. Whenever we share with others that hematology/oncology is what we have chosen to pursue, "I don't know how you can do it, it is just so emotionally draining" is the frequent response. But, that is just it. We have tapped into what moves our hearts. We have sought to build our hopes on things eternal, and eternal inspiration comes from within.

This is a reflection that may influence or inspire the reader to act or think differently when it comes to defining what it means to be accomplished in a competitive, demanding professional environment. This very publication may not be perceived as being as "successful" as the groundbreaking clinical publication with outcomes that change practice. However, if we reach just one professional then we have succeeded, because that is what we set out—that is, what *we* expected—to do.

1. Fuhs DW, Melby MJ, Vejraska MT, Botticelli JT, Davis SL, Pfeiffer DL. The expectation conundrum: Reflections from a residency class. Am J Health Syst Pharm 2011;68:354–6.

Sales in Pharmacy Practice

Valerie Azzopardi Coppenrath, Pharm.D., BCPS
Resident

M y parents have four children. Their oldest and youngest children were born with a passion for business and marketing, while the two middle children (myself included) demonstrated a love for the sciences. We used to tease one another around the dinner table about these differences, which were apparent even in our early career choices. My younger brother Nicholas was promoted rapidly in his position at Central Michigan University calling alumni to solicit donations, while I quit my new position as a cashier at Best Buy to avoid selling Product Replacement Plans at the register. Naturally, my sales-oriented siblings tried to sell me on the advantages of careers in business (fewer years of education, the potential for higher salaries earlier after graduation, and bonuses based on performance). However, I was never quite comfortable with the idea of trying to convince customers that they needed a particular product or service. Of course, it was not in my nature to try to convince my siblings of my point of view. Instead, I would think to myself, *"That's just not me!"*

I completed my doctor of pharmacy degree and started my first position as a pharmacy practice resident in a large, tertiary care teaching hospital on the East Coast. On my internal medicine rotation, most of my early recommendations were generally accepted without much discussion: add an aspirin, titrate insulin doses, and switch captopril to lisinopril or metoprolol tartrate to metoprolol succinate before discharge. I was beginning to grow confident as a new practitioner, and I had even started to enjoy my time in the hospital, which I had previously only viewed as a means to an end in a PGY2 residency in ambulatory care.

One cool October morning, I was discussing a particular patient with the second-year medical resident on my internal medicine team. The patient was a 22-year-old male who had experienced an asthma attack despite having medium-dose inhaled corticosteroids on his active med list. We had discussed this patient in earnest on rounds, discussing nonadherence or inappropriate inhaler technique as potential contributors to the attack. After rounds, I obtained his refill history from his outpatient pharmacy and determined that his past 3 months of refills were on time. I stopped in my office to pick up a metered dose inhaler demonstrator and a spacer and headed back up to the floor. That is when I ran into the second-year resident, Dr. Thayer, on my way to the patient's room. I provided a brief update on my progress and outlined my plan to assess technique and offer a spacer if appropriate. The resident was busy, but she managed a smile and a quick thank-you for my efforts. As I was walking away, I said, "And if technique isn't an issue, we could always consider switching him to Advair." Behind me, I heard her scoff. "I NEVER prescribe Advair," she said, in a condescending tone. "With the black boxed warning and all." I stopped in my tracks, not only because of the sudden change in her demeanor but also because I had absolutely no idea what she was talking about. I turned around but was not able to hide my consternation. She said curtly, "It increases risk of death," before returning to her documentation.

After interviewing our patient, I retreated to the clinical pharmacy office to regroup. Surely my professors at Wayne State University had not led me astray! I pulled the package insert and located the trial it referenced. I printed a copy and sat down with an iced coffee, the way most people would sit down with a newspaper. Perhaps it was the caffeine, but my heart started to race as my conclusions started to form. As I finished, I felt both relieved and full of dread.

One of the medications contained in Advair, when used alone in patients with asthma, was associated with an increased risk of asthma-related death. The patients who received both medications had improved outcomes. So, I was not wrong to recommend Advair as step-up therapy. But, I needed to try and sell my conclusions to Dr. Thayer.

The next day on rounds, I could barely concentrate. My mouth was dry, my palms were sweaty, and the article in my lab coat pocket felt like it added an extra 10 pounds. I was so distracted that I barely noticed rounds coming to an end. Everyone started off in different directions, and I knew my window of opportunity was closing. *"Why do I sound like a mouse?,"* I thought to myself, as I called out the medical resident's name and tried to catch up.

"I looked into that thing that you mentioned yesterday." She stared at me blankly. "About Advair increasing risk of death?" Pause. I waited, wondering if I should repeat myself. After what seemed like an eternity, recognition and then annoyance flickered in her eyes. "Oh, right. Weren't you on rounds? He's being discharged on Flovent." She was already engrossed in another patient's chart. "I know," I stammered. "It's just that...I mean...it might come up again..." I cleared my throat and managed to squeak out my explanation. I could barely follow it myself. "Here, I brought you a copy of the trial. I highlighted the most important parts for you." She continued her documentation. My heart was beating louder than the telemetry machines. I laid it carefully on the counter next to her. I mumbled something about dry powder inhalers and combination medications increasing adherence, but I could not tell if she was still listening. As I walked away, I considered hiding around the corner to see if she took the article with her. I decided I could not handle the potential rejection.

That was the first of many uncomfortable encounters throughout the year. With more practice, I began to figure out which recommendations would be more controversial and would require more research and preparation. One of my co-residents, a PGY2 in infectious diseases, revealed to me that he always tried to discuss controversial or complicated recommendations with the resident before rounds, when there is a little more time and a little less at stake (for both parties). My preceptors trained me in the SBAR method of communication— Situation, Background, Assessment, and Recommendation. I prepared visual aids to bring to rounds—charts of potassium levels and chemical structures of loop diuretics—whatever would strengthen my recommendations. By June, my confidence, delivery, and "recommendation accepted" rate had improved significantly. However, I never really overcame the sick feeling in my stomach during rounds and waited for the 30th with bated breath. I was eager to kiss rounds goodbye and say hello to my own patient visits in the primary care clinics as a PGY2 resident in ambulatory care. *"Patients will be much easier to deal with,"* I kept telling myself.

And for the most part, they were. I was responsible for both chronic disease management and medication therapy management.

Most patients just needed a little help—someone to explain the instructions for each medication, offer ways to save money, or tell how to manage side effects. Most patients were invested in their own care, and the ones who were not often "no-showed" their scheduled appointments. Lester Goodrich was not like most patients.

He was a friendly gentleman referred to me for management of his uncontrolled type 2 diabetes. At our first visit, he smiled and nodded and was able to repeat back my instructions verbatim. Before he left, he asked me for a refill on his Viagra prescription. I reminded him that Dr. Berkowicz had asked me to adjust only his diabetes medications, but I offered to pass along the message regardless. Lester never missed a follow-up visit. I did not find out he was nonadherent until his girlfriend Sandy came to an appointment and ratted him out. Not skipping a beat, I switched gears.

The next 30 minutes were exasperating. I asked about side effects and copayments and his daily schedule. No issues. Sandy laid out all of his medications for him each day and took care of all of his medication refills. Since he was always able to recite his medication regimens with a twinkle in his eye, comprehension did not appear to be an issue. Sandy and I both voiced our concerns about damage to his nerves, eyes, and kidneys, and he just nodded with a smile in the corner of his mouth. That visit ended with his empty promise to take his medicine—and another request for a Viagra refill.

And so it continued. We repeated this elaborate dance every few weeks, and the outcome was always the same. I hoped Sandy and I would eventually wear him down, but I also worried that June 30th might come first. One day I bumped into Dr. Berkowicz in the hallway between exam rooms and apologized for my repeated refill requests for Lester's Viagra. "He hasn't quite grasped the idea that we are supposed to be focusing on his diabetes."

"Oh, no worries," he responded with a professional smile. "It's all part of the job." He walked a few more steps and pulled his next patient's encounter form from the door. He made a few notes and then looked up at me again. "The irony is that his uncontrolled diabetes and blood pressure are likely contributing to his erectile dysfunction." He disappeared into an exam room before I could hug him. *"Bingo!"*

I looked forward to Lester's next appointment like it was a weekend without staffing or being on-call. This time, I was the one with a twinkle in my eye, and I finally got a reaction out of him: "You mean those things are related?"

"They might be. Are you willing to give it a try?" He leaned forward, clapped his hands, and rubbed them together in earnest. "Okay, Doc. Whatever you say!"

I will never forget these experiences. They have helped me realize that the act of "selling" is vital to the effective practice of pharmacy. Whenever I make a recommendation to a prescriber, I am essentially trying to change his mind. Whenever I counsel a patient on a new medication, I am trying to convince her that the potential benefits outweigh the potential risks. Even now, as an assistant professor of pharmacy practice, I am selling my point of view whenever I make a suggestion during a department meeting and whenever I provide constructive feedback on student assignments. Realizing this has prompted me to spend time sharpening my communication skills in addition to my pharmacotherapy skills, and I encourage all pharmacists to consider doing the same. Find out what motivates your audience. Is your patient most concerned about side effects or cost? Determine the best form of communication. Would that recommendation be best delivered in person during a busy clinic block or via e-mail? And finally, communicate clearly and concisely. How much background is needed to orient your audience to the situation? Are you requesting action? What can *you* do to make implementing this suggestion easy?

I never could have imagined that pursuing a career in pharmacy would lead me right back to the type of experiences I had been trying to avoid. But what surprises me most is how much selling in pharmacy practice suits me, after all.

Becoming

Louis L. Bystrak, Pharm.D., BCPS, BCOP
Clinician

Why is it that the characteristics easiest for us to identify in a person, or pharmacist, are the ones we do not want to possess? This was apparent to me as early as orientation to college, and there were plenty of reminders along the way. There still are. In weaker moments, these characteristics can shake your confidence, strike at your motives. These potential pitfalls have manifested themselves in many people, from the pharmacists who loved their job so much they decided to marry it to the dispensers who would have liked nothing more than to divorce their profession altogether but retain the lifestyle it provided. Another common type was the burnt-out professional who knew how everything should be done, but had not the first clue of how to get the ball of *real* change rolling. And there were the hubristic drug authorities who loved to reside high above but who were ignorant of the potential fall that could come from a change in their organization's structure, thus eliminating their position, or the fall that could result from a medication error precipitated by prideful carelessness or overconfidence. There are more examples, but dwelling on them is something I prefer to avoid. Suffice it to say, I recognized, early on, certain toxic behaviors I would have to avoid in the pharmacist I was becoming.

The tricky thing about defining ourselves by what we are not, and hope not to be, is that our cup is still empty. This is certainly a recipe for a hollow and likely abbreviated career path in any field. So, along the way in our education, we get to go shopping for personality traits, career viewpoints, and political agendas that might complement the nuts and bolts, the raw facts that we take from classes, residencies, and fellowships in the hope of building a pharmacy paragon.

For me, balance was the first clearly indispensable building block, both within and between the workplace and private life. Balancing pharmacy with the demands of a personal life is no small task. The preceptors I admire most of all found a balance that worked for them.

They seemed to have a rule about running in life: do not. They were never rushed; they were always poised and peaceful. And all of that was deliciously contagious. They had family, friends, beliefs, hobbies, and smiles. But what amazed me even more was the balance they struck in the workplace. The degree of change that pharmacy has undergone in the past decade and that it will continue to undergo appears to be greater than in some other fields: from the education process to reimbursement to managing patients more independently— reaching from the community to the laboratory. All of these stressors are just waiting to push a pharmacist off the beam. In my training, the preceptors who stood out as role models were the ones who were able to see and balance all of these forces yet remain able to set the patient in front of them as the first priority. This was the balance I decided I would strive to achieve.

Knowledge was next. Not doses and guidelines, but knowledge of the pharmacy world they occupied and of themselves. My models knew what they were capable of, how to go about it, and if it was worth the cost. They did not always verbalize all of this as it was happening because it occurred in their minds too quickly. It was in their explanation afterward that, in passing, it all became clear. More so, they understood the intricacies and egos involved in the health care hierarchy and patient management team. If patient care or patient satisfaction was at stake, they would not hesitate to act swiftly and purposefully. In less acute instances, they would attempt to bring about policy change after convincing management of the necessity of a desired program and the dangers of its absence. Their managing of obstacles was based on their own strengths and their knowledge of the nuances of the situation. It was this non-book-based knowledge that I found most tantalizing.

What was most intoxicating was the gentle touch behind all of this well-balanced knowledge of the pharmacy world. The pharmacists who entranced me the most always approached their work as servants and their profession with a healthy dose of humility. They were not pushovers to aggressive practitioners or aggressive students. They were firm when they had to be, but they never acted like they thought of themselves as more than they were. I think this went along largely with their sense of balance. In short, they realized that they were both always a teacher and always a student.

If I were to build the archetype of a pharmacist, I would start with balance, knowledge, and humility. Perhaps someone is reading this and scoffing at the naive and overly simplistic view. That is fine. All I ask is not to let that disagreement determine your perspective. It is not what we do not want to become that should drive us, but rather, what we desire to be. In the end, I only hope that I am becoming the type of pharmacist that will help build my profession into something I can be proud of and that, in return, the profession will be proud of me.

Celebrating Pharmacy

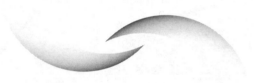

*Joy, rather than happiness, is the goal of life,
for joy is the emotion which accompanies our
fulfilling our natures as human beings. It is
based on the experience of one's identity as a
being of worth and dignity.*

Rollo May

*There lives the dearest freshness deep
down things.*

Gerard Manley Hopkins

My Hopes for Friends and Scholars

Karl Ruch, Pharm.D., BCPS
Clinician/Preceptor

Make us worthy, Lord, to serve our fellow men throughout the world who live and die in poverty and hunger. Give them through our hands this day their daily bread, and by our understanding love, give peace and joy.

–Mother Teresa

Everyone must work to live, but the purpose of life is to serve and to show compassion and the will to help others. Only then have we ourselves become true human beings.

–Albert Schweitzer

Why is the only dream I can dream the dream of giving something beautiful to this overflowing world?

–Linford Detweiler

I have never been so glad to see spring. The season is always extraordinarily beautiful in our Appalachian town of Asheville. However, after 6 interminable months of sick children at home, a slew of spontaneous and severe snow-days (more often than not, translating to "snow-ins" at the hospital), and the usual dreary drab gray-brown of the half-year-hibernating landscape, I relish the scent, sight, and sound of the blooming and waking world like never before. I have historically hated spring, its being the harbinger of that dread season summer, which, during a decade of living in the sweltering Piedmont, had pummeled my subconscious into an overheated hatred of the months usually adored by reasonable people.

But now things are different. The mountain air and spirit of my new hometown has transformed what was heretofore a dreaded season into a time of great excitement and anticipation. And it occurs to me that part of what I love about spring nowadays is that it is a conclusion of things, academically speaking. Hope is in the air: it began a delicate and uncertain seedling with the students' arrival in the fall and then matured in stature and tenacity through the challenges of the year; now, its fragrance fills the April atmosphere with optimism, confidence, and an invigorating sense of accomplishment and freedom.

Ever since I first set foot on my college campus nearly 20 years ago, I have loved academia. Perhaps it was the leathery feel of the old book bindings, the brittle sound of chalk on the board, the oaky smell of professors' pipe tobacco, the perceived autonomy to philosophize until the morning light, and then the laughable panic of waking up 10 minutes after the great bell had sounded for morning classes…: all were an intoxicating blend of novel and mysterious experiences that spoke deeply to my soul. So deeply, in fact, that all this time later, after college, careers, marriage, mortgages, children, *more* school, *more* children…, I still mark my year's beginning in August and its end in May, and why? For many precious and idyllic years, I lived under the tutelage of professors who teach "not to dictate or to profess a discipline or a body of knowledge as much as they are to gladly seek and gladly learn together with their students."[1] This vision inspired not only a love of learning and hope for a life imbued with meaning, but also a sense of gratitude and feeling of generosity that now manifest in me a desire to inspire others and to pass on that sense of hope.

So students have become a great passion in my life, and graduation has become a time of profound celebration. During my last student's final evaluation a few days ago, I found myself positively ebullient with the breathtaking realization that in a few hours, she, having successfully completed all of her requirements for the school, would literally be driving into a completely new adventure, equipped with all that we had happily given her and blessed with our well-wishes. Another former student who has worked several years in the community just wrote to share the thrilling news that through a serendipitous mix of timing, letters, interviews, and dreaming (not to mention her formidable talent and character), she was headed back home to complete a residency and achieve a new vision for her career and family. Reflecting on the year, and realizing what an honor it has been to once again learn and live with such excellent people, I remember something C.S. Lewis once wrote:

It is a serious thing to live in a society of possible gods and god-desses, to remember that even the dullest and most uninterest-ing person you can talk to may one day be a creature which, if you saw it now, you would be strongly tempted to worship.... There are no ordinary people. You have never talked to a mere mortal. Nations, cultures, arts, civilizations—these are mortal, and their life is to ours as the life of a gnat. But it is immortals whom we joke with, work with, marry, snub, and exploit—im-mortal horrors or everlasting splendors.[2]

As the dear students leave and enter into their glittering and per-haps glorious futures, I find myself hoping things for them; spring is a good time to hope. I hope they will find a *home*, a place both sacred and mundane where they can work and play and put into use the many gifts they have been given. I hope they will learn to *rest*, now being the masters of their own schedule after these many years of dreaded deadlines and relentless requirements.

I hope they will now become *mentors*, continuing the cycle of passing knowledge on to the next generation, and yet I also hope they will forever seek to find mentors for themselves. It was St. Ber-nard who said that "he who constitutes himself his own director, be-comes the disciple of a fool." I remember that I foolishly have not only lost the way at times, but also the memory of where I was even going in the first place; I remember, too, the role of mentors, who gave grace to me in those times with notes of encouragement, office visits, coffee chats, and an overwhelming concern for the balance of my life and the peace of my soul. There was the day that my mentor and I had planned to discuss our drug research, but instead, we went to get espresso, and she spent the hours asking questions about my fam-ily and my artistic aspirations. During a season of great inner tumult when I was endlessly debating whether the time was right to start having children, another professor let me hold her 6-month-old during a committee meeting; his brilliant smile and her encouraging words convinced me that the time was indeed right. And then there was that seminal moment when my college mentor attended my senior orches-tral performance one night and my thesis defense the next morning; he has ever since reminded and encouraged me that the left brain is not at odds with the right (or the heart). Now, at the end of another year, having been a guide, teacher, and counselor for another set of my own students, I hope that my friends, and now fellow-sojourners, will have the humility and bravery not only to continue to look for new mentors, but to become mentors as well.

Lastly, and most importantly, I hope my students will learn to *serve*. In the classroom and the clinic, from the 101s to the ICUs, we at every turn have endeavored to instill a sense of servanthood in our young scholars. Caring for others was indeed the very thing that brought most of them to the profession in the first place. But now they are venturing out into the bigger world, and it will be a challenge to remember that the grand armamentarium of knowledge that we have given them was for the purpose of healing and care. As one who reads every white paper and position statement about the future of the profession with equal parts exhilaration and anxiety, I recall to myself the words of Jesus of Nazareth, "look at the birds, free and unfettered, not tied down by a job description, careless in the care of God,"[3] and my hope for myself, and for the fledgling pharmacists, is that we will hear in all of the chaos the words of Mother Teresa and simply remember to *serve* our fellow men and women.

This idea of service is nothing new: one might even say it has been written on the hearts of humankind. Throughout our varied histories and heritages, those of the healing professions have ever found a calling and a commonality in that classic and poetic line from Hippocrates: "In purity and according to divine law will I carry out my life and my art."[4] And for my part, the fountainhead of this desire to serve has been rediscovered in the stories of my youth. There is one story, which, in the circle of relationships that frames my life, is told every spring in purposed proximity to Easter. You may know it:

When James and John, the sons of Zebedee, were seeking to be rewarded with power and position for their discipleship, Jesus told them:

> You've observed how godless rulers throw their weight around... and when people get a little power how quickly it goes to their heads. It's not going to be that way with you. Whoever wants to be great must become a servant. Whoever wants to be first among you must be your slave.[3]

About 10 years ago, up in the valleys of the Blue Ridge Mountains, away from that thick, drowsy, endless summer heat of the Piedmont, I spent a week with a big rowdy crowd of hippies. I have gone back many times since, and I love these people. They are artists: insane, absurdly dressed, egomaniacal, mostly convinced that life's ills are best treated with the brandishing of crystals and the application of poetry, famously undependable..., and I adore them. We had gathered, like birds of a feather, so the saying goes, to learn about singing, writing, playing, and the deeper things that pull us, as humans, not only to each other, but also within, farther in, to our truest selves. I was taking a songwriting class with Bob Franke, the hero of my heroes of many years. As the first class began, I looked apprehensively at my fellow students (of which there were only two) and thought: *surely, I cannot survive a week in such intimacy and immediacy to such a master of my art as this!* Bob began his teaching with a series of songs, including one of my favorites of all time, which includes the verse:

Some say that God is a lover, some say it's an endless void
Some say both, some say she's angry, some say he's just annoyed
But if God felt a hammer in the palm of his hand
Then God knows the way we feel
And love lasts forever
Forever and for real[5]

This was the moment of truest inspiration: the moment when my hope and vision for my life as a healer and an artist expanded to include the serving of another as the ultimate goal. What I learned from Bob that week is that we write to find ourselves, yes, but that we also write because we have an ethical obligation as artists to serve our community, to help our friends and enemies. In the broader picture of my life as a pharmacist, it became clear that we have an ethical obligation as healers to serve our community as well, no matter how commonplace the context, and no matter how considerable the cost. It is what the sons of Zebedee hadn't quite figured out yet, though one can hope and even imagine that they finally did. And that is a hope that I cling to desperately—that they finally realized (and that *I* will finally realize) that being a human means being a leader, yet a leader who washes feet and does the dishes and works with a hammer and gives his or her life away in the service of those in need.

This is my greatest hope for you, dear students: that as leaders, you will learn to serve.

1. Davidson College. Circling the Fountain. Davidson, NC: Davidson College Alumni Association, 1995.
2. Lewis CS. The Weight of Glory and Other Addresses. San Francisco: Harper, 2001.
3. Peterson E. The Message: The Bible in Contemporary Language. Colorado Springs: NavPress, 2003.
4. National Library of Medicine. The Hippocratic Oath. Available at www.nlm.nih.gov/hmd/greek/greek_oath.html. Accessed September 1, 2011.
5. Franke B. Lyric excerpt from the song "Forever." Flying Fish, 1986.

Leave Them Just a Little Different

Charles D. Ponte, Pharm.D., BSc, DPNAP, FAPhA, FASHP, FCCP
Educator/Clinician

In October 2008, when I received the Board of Advisors Award for Excellence in Teaching from the West Virginia University School of Pharmacy, I was asked to deliver a last lecture in which I would espouse my philosophy of teaching. Here are some excerpts and embellishments from that lecture on insights regarding the art of teaching, garnered from 30 years as a didactic and experiential instructor at a large university-based medical center.

There is no greater accolade than to be recognized by your peers and colleagues for your efforts in "doing what you love" and "doing what you were born to do." Sophia Loren was purported to say, "Everything you see, I owe to spaghetti." This statement has meaning to me given my Italian heritage (along with French) and love of pasta. Although I cannot honestly link my academic successes entirely to pasta, everything you see is the sum total of a diet rich in hard work, perseverance, support, mentorship, and, yes, even luck.

I have always enjoyed teaching. In fact, my first recollection of "teaching" others occurred when I was a seventh-grade student at Slocum Grammar School in Waterbury, Connecticut (my hometown).

One night before school, I had gone out with my father in the backyard, flashlight in hand, to search for big game, namely the elusive earthworm or "night crawler." I managed to "bag" a rather large and fat specimen, and I kept him alive in an old soup can filled with dirt. You see, earlier, I had told my seventh-grade teacher that I would bring in the worm and dissect it in front of the class for all to observe. The next morning, earthworm in hand—or should I say earthworm in "can"—I went to school full of anticipation.

Once I had laid bare the internal machinery of the earthworm, all the kids in class came by to look. I provided a short description of what they saw lying pinned to the bottom of a paraffin-filled metal tray. My foray into teaching had begun.

I view myself mainly as a clinician/educator. It's important to note that being an effective clinician also means being a good teacher. In fact, the word *doctor* comes from the Latin *doctus*, a teacher, or *docere*, to teach. Therefore, doctors of pharmacy, doctors of philosophy, or doctors of medicine can be viewed as teachers of their respective disciplines.

Some people are born teachers; their ability to articulate, simplify concepts, and make learning fun is innate and conferred by a higher source. The rest of us have to learn the skills that will enhance our teaching effectiveness and then put them into practice. I have never forgotten the expression "Teaching helps you understand." I used to keep it on a bulletin board next to my desk. Perhaps Einstein said it best: "If you can't explain it simply, you don't understand it well enough."

As an educator, I have strived to be creative and innovative. However, and more importantly, I do not try to be someone I am not.

When I enter a classroom or other educational venue, I don't leave who I am at the door and try to become somebody else. My personality (including the quirks) is enmeshed with my lectures and is an integral part of any dialogue I have with students. I try to engage the audience and make them participate in the learning experience. I made a promise to myself long ago that if I ever became a teacher, I would never bore the audience. I have tried to live up to that promise. I want the learner to "feel" different when he or she leaves the classroom or the patients' bedside from when he/she entered. In other words, a little bit of me is left behind after one of my presentations.

Over the years, I have used various techniques to engage the audience. For small group presentations, I often call on people by name and pose questions or clinical scenarios for them to consider. I never belittle a participant or downplay an answer or response. My goal is to encourage learning, not discourage it. I have also had the learners randomly pick topics (written on small pieces of paper) from an Erlenmeyer flask. In this situation, the audience has no advance notice regarding the topics to be discussed, which encourages spontaneity and the need to "think on your feet." I have even divided groups into teams and held competitions using clinical scenarios or cases as the modus operandi. I also try to capture awkward or uncomfortable moments during the lecture or discussion and put a humorous face on them. Again, I do not publicly embarrass the student, but I always (or at least try to) catch up with the student and thank him/her for being a "good sport." Letting the students witness your vulnerable or humorous side goes a long way toward establishing a positive rapport with the class. They will realize quickly that you're not an "academic stiff" but that, instead, you have human flaws and traits just like them.

The large classroom setting poses many challenges for class engagement. Again, I try to incorporate the same techniques as noted previously for small discussion groups. Importantly, know the room and the technology. Spending the first 10–15 minutes to get the audiovisual equipment up and running is a sure way to lose the audience. In this setting, you have to be more mobile, let the audience see you, and not hide behind the podium. Unless amplified, you also have to project your voice so they can hear you. Proper enunciation/pronunciation and variable voice pitch also go a long way toward ensuring a successful presentation. Remember, your voice will make or break you. The large classroom often favors the use of PowerPoint as the instructional mode of choice. If this instructional method is used, I purposely avoid "busy," difficult-to-read slides and limit the use of imbedded "bells and whistles," which may distract from and negatively affect learning.

In the patient care environment, I am a strong proponent of emulating the behaviors I want my students to master. It's important for the student to see me conduct a good drug history, effectively counsel a patient, and provide consultation and instruction to other health care providers. At the bedside, I want them to see me provide comfort, a hand to hold, or an ear to listen to a patient in need of human empathy and compassion. However, this up-close-and-personal approach can backfire. You may find yourself sitting on the bed of someone with urinary incontinence, as I did during pharmacy teaching rounds. At least this teaches the students a valuable lesson—be careful where you sit.

Earlier, I mentioned the use of PowerPoint presentations. I learned early on that students don't want or particularly like someone who simply reads off his or her PowerPoint slides or notes from a textbook. If that's a professor's modus operandi, then it should be no surprise when students choose not to attend class. Why should a student attend when everything he/she needs to know (for the exam) has already been provided? I believe students should want to come to my class or presentation because they're interested in learning about my "take" on the subject matter. How have I been able to filter the information through my own experiences and knowledge and apply it to real-world situations in a meaningful and practical way? Students may not be hungry for knowledge itself but for the *application* of knowledge. Today's college-age learner, who wants to be entertained, perhaps unknowingly expects his/her professors to have perfected some kind of "standup" routine.

If you want to be an effective educator, learn to be flexible, and adapt to changing situations in the classroom or (for that matter) at the patient's bedside. Remember, a strong desire and interest in teaching is necessary if you are to become an effective conveyor of messages. Seek out teaching opportunities beyond your daily professional responsibilities, and strive to improve your teaching proficiency. Observe good teachers (think back on your past teachers or professors, preceptors or speakers from recent meetings or symposia). Adapt some of their techniques to your own style of instruction.

One of the best teachers I ever had was named Tom Hall. He taught at Crosby High School located in downtown Waterbury, Connecticut. Mr. Hall was my homeroom teacher, and he taught freshman Latin and English. Well, it wasn't until I took first-year Latin from him that I realized what a special teacher he was. Simply put, he brought the subject to life. He exuded passion for his subject and his craft. He was eloquent, moving about the front of the class, using expressive hand gestures to make points, and exhibiting booming voice projection together with exquisite enunciation and pronunciation of the spoken word. Appearance was also important to Mr. Hall. He was clearly one of the best-dressed faculty at the school. He even wore a black carnation on his sport coat lapel during the Ides of March, when Julius Caesar was assassinated in 44 BC. It was his way of paying homage to the fallen leader. Mr. Hall embodied the attributes that separate good teachers from great teachers: enthusiasm, total command of the subject matter, excellent communication skills, passion, and the ability to turn the lecture into a living, breathing organism. You could see the twinkle in his eyes when he lectured to the class.

At this point, it's important to mention that no personal or professional accomplishments or successes occur in a vacuum, devoid of outside influences. Likewise, teaching success is the sum total of various factors (some alluded to in my earlier remarks)—namely, innate ability, passion, a strong knowledge base, a commitment to self-betterment, student respect, and a willingness to experiment with novel or untapped instructional methods and technologies.

With few exceptions, successful individuals have a strong work ethic and don't procrastinate. Mark Twain once said, "Never put off until tomorrow what you can do the day after tomorrow." This is not sound advice for the person who wants to be a successful educator. A strong work ethic is difficult to learn or instill, but if recognized, it should be nurtured and allowed to grow. Policies/procedures and other initiatives must be in place in the work setting to guarantee success. The idea of mentorship has been addressed in many publications, and its importance to your success (even in teaching) should never be underestimated.

Many years ago, Joan Mullin wrote an article titled "Philosophical Backgrounds for Mentoring the Pharmacy Professional," in which she mentions how the mentor provides the "lore of the field" and passes along "practical wisdom." What a meaningful statement! An individual with a mentor who can share his/her professional "street smarts" is indeed fortunate. This is so important, yet we rarely take advantage of the collective teaching wisdom in our schools and actively seek teaching mentors. Finally, and most importantly, emotional support during your career is crucial. Seek the people and/or institutions that can share in your triumphs and failures. Such support will encourage steadfastness of purpose and greater accomplishments.

The distinguished poet and activist Maya Angelou said, "I've learned that people will forget what you said, people will forget what you did, but people will never forget how you made them feel." When you leave the classroom or the patient's bedside, leave the students feeling just a little different about their profession, their knowledge, and themselves.

Beauty in Change

Joel Henneberry, Pharm.D. Candidate 2012
Student

I know the life of the student pharmacist—the subtleties, the frustrations, the losses, and the victories. I know the struggle to divulge, digest, and present intangible health information. I know the obsession with accuracy, safety, and gray-world validity. I know that somewhere between 2006 and 2012, I will have matured into a member of the most accessible health care profession. I know it is my task to translate knowledge into healing every time I put on the white coat. But it is what I do not know that excites me most— what it would feel like to stand up for the patient when his or her best interest has been lost in the system, what it would feel like to interact with the health care team, and what it would mean to me to put clinical pharmacy into action for the benefit of my patients.

My journey of maturation had a peculiar start—in the distant past. As a pre-pharmacy student at the St. Louis College of Pharmacy, I dove into the history of pharmacy, touching the pages of books 100 and 200 years my senior. The archives revealed that pharmacy is a profession accustomed to constant change. With time, I watched the magic of medication evolve into science, the compounding druggist evolve into the care-guiding pharmacist, and the bread-and-butter customer evolve into the cornerstone patient. At times, there was a great jostling between the health professions as written and unwritten boundaries were crossed and turfs, guarded. At times, the future looked bleak for pharmacy, with health information seemingly withheld from the very patients it was meant to heal. At times, the prospect of technological advance, first in manufacturing and later in robotics, seemed to condemn the livelihood of pharmacists everywhere, as if to label them obsolete. With each advance, every generation of pharmacists made necessary changes and met challenges considered insurmountable. The profession persisted until even the lofty goal of reimbursement for cognitive services was obtained in the undisputed form of Medication Therapy Management, the crowning accomplishment of almost a century of sweat spent toward that end.

And here, I arrived abruptly in the present, burning with excitement for a profession as though I was its biggest fan. Fresh from the white coat ceremony at the Chase Park Plaza Hotel on Lindell Boulevard, I saw my opportunity to join the ranks becoming a reality. But by no means was the charted course easy—every letter grade was an earned badge, every examination a door to be unlocked, every day a lap in the yearly marathon of higher learning at the College. Much as my white coat did not emerge from the pharmaceutics laboratory in its originally immaculate condition, my classroom achievement did not reflect the intellect I thought I possessed when I began. The curriculum of pharmacy school has reached a level of difficulty capable of humbling some of the greatest minds of my generation (among whom I stake no claim, though I certainly sat beside them in class), requiring incredible discipline and an athletic mind. The more I experienced outside the classroom, the more I realized that school was just a sampling before the feast, only a warm-up lap before the sprint.

When I saw clinical pharmacy take the form of a pharmacy practice professor working at the John Cochran division of the Veterans Affairs Medical Center in St. Louis, I knew the future of pharmacy was bright. I saw him interact with an acute care team of providers, perfectly filling his niche as a medication expert, educating medical residents, student pharmacists, and patients; recommending therapies to attendings; and monitoring efficacy, interactions, and adverse effects, all in the same afternoon. Rounding with the team was exciting! And VA clinical pharmacists sign a scope of practice agreement to receive mid-level prescribing rights? I had to see more of this venue of pharmacy.

After my second professional year of study, I was fortunate to be accepted into the VALOR program at the VA, where I spent my summer shadowing staff and clinical pharmacists at John Cochran and Jefferson Barracks. I loved every day. I was enthralled with the workhorse of VA technology called CPRS, or Computerized Patient Record System. All members of the health care team could interface with the patient's charts electronically, remotely view x-rays, see the trends in laboratory results, and recommend and receive orders for consultation. With test results so readily available, pharmacists could translate all that is Pharm.D. into practical and astute recommendations and, in so doing, guide therapy toward effectiveness and farther from risk. Even the "staff" pharmacists at the VA fulfilled "clinical" roles as they worked with each veteran at discharge and for refills. The electronic charts permitted efficient verification of the facts and supported the making of enlightened clinical decisions.

The beauty was in the teamwork that coordinated comprehensive patient care. A consult to a physical therapist was sandwiched between a nurse practitioner's recommendations and a note from the chaplain's services about the religious preferences of the patient. An ambulatory care pharmacist accepted a consult to become the primary provider of a diabetic patient's chronic disease state management, and another clinical pharmacist rounded earlier that day with the infectious disease team, guiding the final touches of therapy for the patient's diabetic foot ulcer, complicated by resistant strains of *Staph. aureus.* The anticoagulation clinic buzzed with pharmacists managing elusive INRs. The critical care pharmacist anchored his team with a resolve equal to the most complex and harrowing cases, day after lifesaving day.

I realize my perspective is highly idealistic. I also realize my current experience is limited. I know reality can be harsh and can seem unyielding. However, I believe the ghosts of pharmacy past would praise the advancement of the profession if they could see us now. We have accomplished so much. We are not only welcomed to the bedside but also invited, because our expertise is vital to high-quality health care. We have not wasted pharmacy's efforts in the earliest ancestors of today's hospitals or in the earliest versions of public health initiatives as embodied in the neighborhood druggist. Our profession has kept stride with the profound advances of health science and is responsible for many of its earliest leaps. Our traditionally timid profession has realized true autonomy in some areas, and the assertive individuals among us continue to push for more, until every patient achieves his/her right to the care of a pharmacist.

As I prepare to ship out to the Indian Health Service in South Dakota for my first of eight 5-week advanced pharmacy practice experiences, I am thrilled to be apprenticed to a profession so accustomed to change. I have great faith in the leaders of pharmacy who push us forward, those who are the groundbreakers in health care reform and who trace the pen of legislation. I yearn to take my place beside the patient and become a vital mediator of health care. I anticipate the day when I might contribute to the vast annals of evidence-based medicine through clinical research. I wonder what shape my career path will take and in which practice environments I will be privileged to participate during my life. Our field is growing and our torch burns bright. More than anything else, change is what makes pharmacy beautiful. Embrace it.

Afterword

Confessing, Searching, Nourishing
William A. Zellmer, B.S. (Pharmacy), M.P.H.

I have a confession.

When Mike Maddux and Tom Zlatic invited me to become coeditor of this book, skepticism complicated my thoughts about the merit of the project. While I recognized the value of a collection of reflective, personal stories by pharmacists who care for patients, I wondered, would there really be enough worthy contributions to fill a book? I knew from my years as a pharmacy journal editor that many pharmacists can write coherently and cogently on technical issues, but I doubted that more than a few had mastered the art of reflective writing—writing that comes from both the head and the heart.

The dominant segment of my brain, which seems to live on a sunny hill alongside a babbling brook, sensed that this book could make an important contribution to the literature of pharmacy, so I agreed to collaborate. There's another part of my brain, a constant presence that is usually kept in check, which hunkers in a dim valley and insists on seeing contingency plans. Yet again, I heard its tiresome refrain, "What will you do if things fall apart?" In this case, the instantaneously formulated backup plan from the overlord on the hill was to look for previously published material that could be repurposed to flesh out the book. Not a great plan, but it put the pest at ease.

Happily, no plan B was required. All of this book's content is original. Many of the authors have benefited from Tom Zlatic's excellent coaching in the art of writing a well-crafted reflection.

I've now corrected my bias about the capacity of pharmacists to think deeply about their professional lives and to write engagingly about learning from their experiences.

The essays in this book have refreshed my view of pharmacy as a thoughtful, animated profession.

....

In 1996, I presented and published a lecture titled, "Searching for the Soul of Pharmacy."[1] Drawing on the writing of Thomas Moore, a psychotherapist, I said that pharmacy cannot become a complete profession unless its practitioners embody "soul" as defined by Moore:

> Soul is not a thing, but a quality or a dimension of experiencing life and ourselves. It has to do with depth, value, relatedness, heart, and personal substance. I do not use the word here as an object of religious belief or something to do with immortality.[2]

In my lecture, I was critical of pharmacists who isolated themselves from patients and who passively accepted a narrow, technical focus in pharmacy practice. I wrote, "People want and need pharmacists...with soul. Let's dedicate ourselves to remaking this occupation of ours into a profession that gives people what they want and need....Each of us must take personal responsibility for making this happen."

In my prescription for "nourishing the soul of pharmacy," I suggested 10 actions in support of this cause. Among the ideas were:

- Recognize and honor pharmacists who have demonstrated an authentic professional commitment to patients. We need more heroes in the frontline ranks of pharmacy.
- Increase efforts to develop and enrich the work of frontline pharmacists in all practice settings. Let's not become distracted from the fact that the true nature of our discipline is defined in the everyday interface between pharmacists and patients.
- Foster a nationwide dialogue among pharmacists and physicians and consumer representatives about the problems related to medication use and what these three groups can do together to make the situation better.

If I were writing that action plan today, I would include the following point near the top of my list:

- Encourage pharmacists to share stories about the "depth, value, relatedness, heart, and personal substance" of their interactions with patients.

The writing in this book puts on display the humanity of pharmacists. The stories show pharmacists who have overcome the fear of taking risks in helping people make the best use of medicines. The writers tell how they have drawn lessons from their successes and failures to give them the will and strength to continue their self-development and mentorship of competent, compassionate, and caring health professionals.

The pharmacists who contributed to this book have shown how to nourish the soul of pharmacy.

....

When one *lives through* a process of gradual change (such as the conversion of an occupation into a profession), as opposed to *observing* change from a distance, it can be difficult to discern the full measure of the emerging new order. The cumulated effects of small, haphazard mutations can be made more apparent if one can find signposts that give a sense of the direction and magnitude of change. One new signal related to pharmacy's transformation recently became apparent to me.

Every year for the past four decades, I have visited a few pharmacy departments in hospitals across the country. It has been a way of staying in touch with the field and helping retain a measure of credibility as a staff member of a pharmacists' association and, now, as a consultant on professional and strategic issues in the profession.

"Show me what you're proudest of."

"Tell me about the major opportunities and challenges you are facing."

These are my requests when I schedule one of my field trips. My hosts' interpretations of my agenda have altered markedly in recent years.

It used to be that I was shown primarily the inner workings of the central pharmacy department—its version of unit dose drug distribution, its compliance with standards for sterile compounding, and the latest automation and technology, with maybe a side trip to a decentralized pharmacy. I was witness to a production culture within the department.[3]

Lately, especially in pharmacies that have residents, my hosts have often skipped the central pharmacy entirely; implicitly, they are telling me, "We have the basic infrastructure of the pharmacy enterprise under control." What I have been shown instead is how pharmacists interact with physicians, nurses, and patients. I have been witnessing a shift to a patient-care culture.

In a recent visit, my tour included observation of a team-meeting of a nurse practitioner, bedside nurses, social workers, and a pharmacist reviewing the status of every patient on an acute-care medicine unit. The pharmacist, integrating knowledge of medicines with first-hand knowledge of the patient, often added information and opinions that influenced the direction of care for a patient.

Increasingly, I have seen evidence of physicians routinely asking the pharmacist to monitor a patient's response to a medicine and adjust the dosage as indicated.

I have heard plans to expand pharmacist-managed clinics, such as for anticoagulation, hyperlipidemia, hypertension, or HIV therapy.

And I have been told stories. For example, one pharmacist described how she found the key to stabilizing a psychotic patient who had been disruptive in the ICU. To the gratitude of the patient, his family, and the ICU team, the pharmacist applied her knowledge and experience in identifying just the right therapy.

Another pharmacist told me how he eased a patient's transition to inpatient care by minimizing switches in her long-stable medication regimen for diabetes. I sensed that this pharmacist had to choose between giving priority to the interests and desires of the patient versus strict compliance with hospital rules, and that he was confident in his decisions.

Firsthand observations and experiences such as these have buttressed in my mind the lessons from the essays in this book, helping me see that today's leading edge in pharmacy is vastly different from what it was not that long ago.

I find in this book's stories a great source of hope for the future of pharmacy as a health profession.

1. Zellmer WA. Searching for the soul of pharmacy. Am J Health Syst Pharm 1996;53:1911–6.
2. Moore T. Care of the Soul: A Guide for Cultivating Depth and Sacredness in Everyday Life. New York: HarperCollins, 1992.
3. Pierpaoli PG. Creatively using our intellectual capital [editorial]. Am J Health Syst Pharm 2009;66:1087.

Appendix I

Reflection as a Learning Strategy

Thomas D. Zlatic, Ph.D.

Many pedagogical approaches use reflective writing as a learning strategy. Because reflective writing is supported by so many different theoretical approaches, can take many forms, and can serve many purposes, an instructor should clarify the intended goals before selecting methods, assignments, and criteria.

Below are some general suggestions for using reflective writing as a learning tool, with particular emphasis on the type of reflective writing contained in this volume.

As students engage in service learning and clinical experiences, they are sometimes asked to keep a journal of reflections. One purpose of such assignments is to expose students to populations outside their normal experiences—the homeless, the elderly, immigrants, abused children, the chronically ill, racial minorities—so that the broadening of their experiences can enhance their potential for empathic patient care.

Journaling alone, however, does not ineluctably lead to insight or enhanced practice. Improvement requires criteria, models, practice, and feedback.

Criteria/Directions

As in any assignment, clear criteria are essential. Because reflection can have various meanings, the instructor must clarify what it means for this particular experience. Criteria should provide a picture of what good practice is and serve as a tool for assessment. Although the criteria should be clear and specific, they should not be confining; rather, they should permit flexibility and creativity. A journal entry is not necessarily equal to the sum of its parts: a holistic evaluation may be more appropriate than a tally of discrete "points." Below is one example of criteria for reflection based on observation, response, analysis, and planning. Each instructor should create/adapt criteria for the specific goals in mind.

1. Observe
   • Accurately and vividly record objective observations of your site experiences (events, people, actions, setting, etc.).

2. Respond
   • Convincingly record subjective responses to your service experiences (thoughts, emotions, values, and judgments).

3. Analyze/Evaluate
   • Find insights, patterns, structure, categories, meanings, causes, effects, and relationships in what you observed and reflected on.
   • Evaluate facts, inferences, and your personal responses, determining the correctness or relative suitability of actions, beliefs, systems, and attitudes.

For example, when appropriate, classify events, people, situations, and responses; infer reasons/motivations/causes for what occurred; identify alternative strategies that might have been performed to improve service. Identify changes in structure or procedure that would improve service. Identify what values/worldviews were operative (yours and those of others). Interpret the behavior of others. Clarify your own values, motivations, goals. Evaluate the effectiveness of self and others.

4. Plan
   • Identify the knowledge, skills, attitudes, and resources needed to be successful.
   • Devise strategies to procure the necessary knowledge, skills, attitudes, resources.
   • Create specific action plans to improve service, both your own and the agency's.
   • Modify action plans as necessary.

The criteria should not be covered sequentially in the reflection, one after the other in separate paragraphs. Rather, guide students to integrate the steps; for instance, blend description and response. In addition, the criteria need not be addressed in the same order. For example, writers might begin with the insight or emotional response and then re-create the experience that led to insight and response.

In addition to criteria, self-assessment questions can help guide writers. Provided to potential contributors to this book were these questions:

- Does the reflection render or dramatize the situation/event (does it "show" rather than "tell" what happened, using detailed, perhaps imaginative description)?
- Does it avoid the obvious—what most practitioners already know?
- Does it avoid sentimentality and clichés ("I just want to make a difference in one person's life")?
- Does it raise new ideas or deepen the reader's thinking on the topic?
- Would the reflection influence or "inspire" the reader to act or think differently?
- Does it promote the value of reflection in a patient-oriented profession?

Instructors also should specify all expectations for the journals—for instance, the number of entries, frequency, length, timetables, format, and medium (electronic, handwritten, hard copy, bound).

Examples
Students should be given examples of reflections that meet the established criteria. To avoid the possibility that students might slavishly follow one format, provide a variety of examples; none should be used as a template. Emphasize individuality and originality.

Exercises
Not all samples of reflection given to students should be excellent. Provide students with three or more examples of varying quality, one at a time. Ask the students to assess individually the journal entry on the basis of the criteria; then, have them discuss and justify their assessments. Follow the same procedure for the other samples so that they can understand and internalize the criteria. If students find that any criteria are not met in a reflection, ask them to rewrite that component of the journal entry.

Feedback

Most importantly, reflection should be dialogic. Continual instructor feedback provides encouragement and challenges to student observations. It is through dialogue, whether written or oral, that students can get a more objective perspective so they can reexamine their values and conclusions.

Students' journal entries can be insightful, moving, and truly inspiring. But not always. Sometimes the entries are incomplete, inaccurate, or superficial; they can reveal immaturity, sociocentricity, and prejudice. This is not unexpected; it is a reason for assigning the journals in the first place.

Each student is an individual, but from the journal responses students provide, some can be categorized into groups. Some students clearly convey that, at their sites, they are tourists. They visit as some Americans do foreign countries: they bring with them the baggage of their own culture and merely skim the surface of the alien culture, sampling but not interiorizing. They marvel at the unusual, dutifully visit important sights, take the required pictures, and write an interesting travelogue, but they return as the same individuals who began the trip. They are broadened but are not challenged or changed by what they encounter.

Worse, some students interpret their sites as freak shows. They are not simply aloof, but mocking. They delight in storytelling that accentuates the bizarre; they ridicule what they cannot understand.

The critics are judgmental. Like the tourists, they hold on to their own perspectives and value systems, but they become even more convinced of the moral superiority of their own positions, from which they condemn those from different backgrounds. Often, without proper intervention, they end the semester with more entrenched prejudices than when they began.

The sentimental do-gooders, however, display a perennially rosy but superficial understanding. They can be identified by hyperbolic platitudes about "wanting to make a difference," which substitute for analysis of complex social issues and human psychology. Often, their sympathy does not blossom into empathy. They feel "for" their clients but not "with" them.

Sometimes, the do-gooder is a tourist or critic in disguise, uttering the types of remarks they think the instructor wants to hear. Frequently, they have too-sudden "conversions," professing to have learned life-changing insights from trivial incidents. Often, these entries are well written—just not convincing.

The goal, of course, is to encourage students to become empathetic practitioners, willing to examine their beliefs and perspectives in light of those of others. We want them to honestly explore values and complex issues beyond conventional platitudes so that they can interact with patients with understanding and empathic care.

The instructor has the potential to guide all of these students toward more complex, humanistic, and empathic responses. But it must be a delicate interaction. The instructor must realize the intrusive nature of the feedback. We ask students to be honest and open as they disclose private, intimate thoughts. By placing their values and opinions on display, they create vulnerability. We must be aware that to be given access to the journal of another person is a privilege. The reviewer's responses cannot be simply analytic. He or she must respond not to a text, but to a person.

Of course, general guidelines for any type of feedback apply. Feedback should be criteria-referenced, performance-based, and student-oriented. Don't criticize the person, but rather, evaluate the performance on the basis of objective criteria, citing particular passages as evidence for the assessment. The feedback should be appropriate to the level and personality of the student. Use the traditional feedback sandwich approach: begin with something positive or complimentary, suggest ways to improve, and conclude with encouragement and confidence in success.

However, given the intimate nature of journaling, other strategies are essential as well.

Students, like all of us, come with biases, prejudices, and misconceptions. Some are uncomfortable or even intolerant regarding issues of race and gender. Some have little experience with those from different backgrounds. Their journal entries can reflect egocentricity and inability to empathize. For instance, students working with abused or abandoned children sometimes become upset with the behavior of clients and staff. Upon encountering 5-year-old children using profane language, they are shocked and indignant, protesting, "If I would have used such language, I would have had my mouth rinsed out with soap." They form or reconfirm stereotypical opinions that are rational—from their own limited backgrounds—but they do not recognize what it means to grow up poor without parents and other role models to inculcate values. They lack the experience and the imagination to recognize that, had they come from such a background themselves, it is likely they would be acting no differently from these children. They cannot empathize because their experience is narrow.

Helping students come to such realizations requires tact. Acknowledge your understanding of how a good and reasonable person might come to such conclusions. Be willing to provide appropriate self-revelation: give an anecdote of how you have reacted in the same way in a similar circumstance; then, provide alternative explanations or reactions. Often, asking questions, a Socratic approach, can be effective. "Why do you think she acted that way?" "Are there other possible explanations for her behavior?" "How is this related to the article we read in class?" "What assumptions lie behind this conclusion?" "Are those assumptions valid?" Try to create situations that lead to "aha" experiences; when old paradigms begin to crumble, fresh insight can take hold.

When possible, avoid judgment but provide facts. Recommend readings (articles or short stories) or films that can re-contextualize the experience. Suggest topics for future journal entries. Tell a pertinent story. Ask the student to write about this experience from the perspective of a patient or caregiver.

Give students the benefit of the doubt. If the student's comments are ambiguous, praise a generous interpretation. Probe to make sure you understand. If a student writes something that should be challenged, sometimes you can pretend to misunderstand: ask the writer to try to be clearer so that a less perceptive reader does not interpret the writer's reaction the wrong way. Humor also can be used to soften criticism, implied or otherwise. Of course, at times, it is important to be direct, but generally, don't lecture or enforce agreement; leave space for students to continue to be honest in their responses and open for growth.

Often, the tone established is as important as what is said. Tone is attitude—attitude toward your audience or topic. Our voices automatically convey tone: surprise, anger, skepticism, indifference, excitement, disapproval, admiration, appreciation, superiority, and thousands of other subtleties—all of these can be conveyed by one spoken word, such as "hello." Tone does not disappear in the silence of writing. The reader imaginatively re-creates tone, based on contextual cues and psychological factors. Content, word choice, sentence structure, examples, and orthographic devices (exclamation points, underlines, CAPS, font color, and font size) help the reader infer tone. But, of course, the reader can reconstruct the wrong tone. We are all sensitive to criticism; particularly when we are being evaluated, we can infer more negativity than the writer intended. The "Dear Mr. Smith" salutations in letters and the emoticons in e-mail are testimony to the need to reassure readers about the friendly tone of the correspondence. In conversation, it is easy to tell whether "you're doing OK" is good-natured praise or a reluctant acknowledgment of bare sufficiency. We insecure readers are likely to infer the latter. Overconfident students might interpret such a comment as an indicator that she does not need to make any improvements. Again, feedback should be student-oriented, so the same tone is not appropriate for each student.

In general, though, given the insecurity of most writers, be sure to provide continual support. Acknowledge good effort and good work; praise, empathize, and encourage. Thank the student for altruistic behavior or for particularly compelling insights.

Feedback should be ongoing. Pick up the journal often, discern patterns and themes, and provide guidance for future work. Although, given privacy issues, peer assessment normally is not appropriate for journal entries, you should require the student to complete periodic self-assessments based on criteria, and then provide feedback to the self-assessment.

More succinctly, when providing feedback, be the empathic, caring practitioner that you want your students to become. Model empathy and care through your feedback. Don't be judgmental, cynical, angry, supercilious, impatient, impersonal, or intimidating. Be open to students and to personal growth. Guide the students in ways to nourish the soul of pharmacy.

Some Resources for Teaching Reflective Writing

Many resources related to reflective writing, including rubrics and assessment forms, are available in print and electronic media.[1] In the tables and boxes below are a few additional resources, including some practice exercises for student.

---

1 For instance, Moon JA. A Handbook of Reflective and Experiential Learning. London: RoutledgeFalmer, 2004. DiRanna K, Osmundson E, Topps J, et al. Assessment-Centered Teaching: A Reflective Practice. Thousand Oaks, CA: Corwin Press, 2008. Bolton G. Reflective Practice: Writing and Professional Development. Los Angeles: Sage, 2010.

Value Rubric for Intercultural Knowledge and Competence

The American Association of Colleges and Universities has published several rubrics for college ability outcome. The following rubric for Intercultural Knowledge and Competence can be helpful when designing outcomes and criteria for reflective journaling.

INTERCULTURAL KNOWLEDGE AND COMPETENCE VALUE RUBRIC

for more information, please contact value@aacu.org

Definition

Intercultural Knowledge and Competence is "a set of cognitive, affective, and behavioral skills and characteristics that support effective and appropriate interaction in a variety of cultural contexts." (Bennett, J. M. (2008). "Transformative training: Designing programs for culture learning." In M. A. Moodian (Ed.), *Contemporary leadership and intercultural competence: Understanding and utilizing cultural diversity to build successful organizations* (pp. 95-110). Thousand Oaks, CA: Sage.)

Evaluators are encouraged to assign a zero to any work sample or collection of work that does not meet benchmark (cell one) level performance.

	Capstone 4	Milestones 3	Milestones 2	Benchmark 1
Knowledge *Cultural self-awareness*	Articulates insights into own cultural rules and biases (e.g. seeking complexity; aware of how her/his experiences have shaped these rules, and how to recognize and respond to cultural biases, resulting in a shift in self-description.)	Recognizes new perspectives about own cultural rules and biases (e.g. not looking for sameness; comfortable with the complexities that new perspectives offer.)	Identifies own cultural rules and biases (e.g. with a strong preference for those rules shared with own cultural group and seeks the same in others.)	Shows minimal awareness of own cultural rules and biases (even those shared with own cultural group(s)) (e.g. uncomfortable with identifying possible cultural differences with others.)
Knowledge *Knowledge of cultural worldview frameworks*	Demonstrates sophisticated understanding of the complexity of elements important to members of another culture in relation to its history, values, politics, communication styles, economy, or beliefs & practices.	Demonstrates adequate understanding of the complexity of elements important to members of another culture in relation to its history, values, politics, communication styles, economy, or beliefs & practices.	Demonstrates partial understanding of the complexity of elements important to members of another culture in relation to its history, values, politics, communication styles, economy, or beliefs & practices.	Demonstrates surface understanding of the complexity of elements important to members of another culture in relation to its history, politics, communication styles, economy, or beliefs & practices.
Skills *Empathy*	Interprets intercultural experience from the perspectives of own and more than one worldview and demonstrates ability to act in a supportive manner that recognizes the feelings of another cultural group	Recognizes intellectual and emotional dimensions of more than one worldview and sometimes uses more than one worldview in interactions	Identifies components of other cultural perspectives but responds in all situations with own worldview	Views the experience of others but does so through own cultural worldview
Skills *Verbal and non-verbal communication*	Articulates a complex understanding of cultural differences in verbal and nonverbal communication (e.g. demonstrates understanding of the degree to which people use physical contact while communicating in different cultures or use direct/indirect and explicit/implicit meanings) and is able to skillfully negotiate a shared understanding based on those differences.	Recognizes and participates in cultural differences in verbal and nonverbal communication and begins to negotiate a shared understanding based on those differences.	Identifies some cultural differences in verbal and nonverbal communication and is aware that misunderstandings can occur based on those differences but is still unable to negotiate a shared understanding.	Has a minimal level of understanding of cultural differences in verbal and nonverbal communication; is unable to negotiate a shared understanding.
Attitudes *Curiosity*	Asks complex questions about other cultures, seeks out and articulates answers to those questions which reflect multiple cultural perspectives	Asks deeper questions about other cultures and seeks out answers to those questions	Asks simple or surface questions about other cultures	States minimal interest in learning more about other cultures
Attitudes *Openness*	Initiates and develops interactions with culturally different others. Suspends judgment in valuing her/his interactions with culturally different others.	Begins to initiate and develop interactions with culturally different others. Begins to suspend judgment in valuing interactions with culturally different others.	Expresses openness to most if not all interactions with culturally different others. Has difficulty suspending any judgment in her/his valuing of interactions with culturally different others, and is aware of own judgment and expresses a willingness to change.	Receptive to interacting with culturally different others. Has difficulty suspending any judgment in her/his interactions with culturally different others, but is unaware of own judgment.

Reprinted with permission from: Assessing Outcomes and Improving Achievement: Tips and Tools for Using Rubrics. Copyright 2010 by the Association of American Colleges and Universities.

A Rubric for Reflection Essays

	Exemplary	Developing	Not Acceptable
Account	Is perceptive. Describes important facts and events that are organized around a main point. Dramatizes the narrative through fresh, concrete, imaginative detail	Organizes the description around a point. Sometimes uses clichés and commonplace images instead of fresh description and perception	Provides mainly a chronological description of events without an apparent framework or purpose. Tells rather than shows what happens. Relies on stereotypical description. Includes irrelevant material
Response	Provides honest and open self-disclosure, displaying appropriate reaction to the situation. Avoids superficial and sentimental responses	Provides honest but reserved self-disclosure. At times, is self-defensive. At times, demonstrates superficial responses	Does not provide self-disclosure or does not provide a convincing response. Manufactures a response to meet instructor expectations
Analysis and insight	Demonstrates awareness of complexity; finds patterns or meanings in events. Connects the experience to course topics or to other areas of personal life. Acknowledges personal values and values of others. Demonstrates a willingness to probe ideas and values	Comes to personal insight but with limited breadth or depth. Connects to other topics but in a limited or artificial way. Does not always acknowledge own values or understand values of others. Demonstrates willingness to probe in some areas	Does not analyze or provides superficial analysis and comes to questionable conclusions. Does not support analysis with course readings and discussions. Does not demonstrate an understanding of the role of values in the situation. Does not move beyond stereotypes
Planning	Correctly assesses one's own strengths/weaknesses regarding the incident; identifies goals for improvement; creates a realistic plan to improve. Follows up on plans and modifies when necessary	Recognizes need for improvement; identifies some goals. Identifies some steps to take to reach the goals. Sometimes follows up on the plans	Does not identify problems or weaknesses. Does not create goals or plans. Creates unrealistic goals or plans. Does not show evidence of implementing plans

Criteria for Reflection on Personal Growth

Some faculty require students to keep journals of their progress on mastering the abilities required for completion of a course or clinical rotation. Faculty can adapt the following criteria to help students develop a self-reflective practice.

- The student chooses for reflection an activity/experience that allows substantive reflection on the abilities being practiced.
- The student adequately details the abilities/learning (i.e., the knowledge, skills, attitudes, and values that are involved in the activity).
- The student insightfully assesses strengths and weaknesses (the focus is not on the activity, but on student performance).
- The student includes a convincing discussion of subjective responses and emotions/attitudes.
- The student accurately assesses his or her level of mastery.
- The student demonstrates breadth and depth of analysis.
- The student in multiple reflections demonstrates longitudinal improvement.
- The student identifies areas for improvement or provides evidence that none is needed.
- The student creates a plan for improvement or further development.
- The writing is clear, organized, and sufficiently developed with convincing evidence/details.

Practice Activities

To help students better understand reflective writing, consider assigning activities such as these.

1. Assess one or more of the reflections in this collection using the criteria above.

2. Rewrite (improve) the observation component of one of the reflections in this collection.

3. Rewrite (improve) the response component of one of the reflections in this collection.

4. Rewrite (improve) the analysis component of one of the reflections in this collection.

5. Rewrite (improve) the planning component of one of the reflections in this collection.

6. Write a reflection in which you extend or come to different conclusions from one of the essays in this collection.

7. Provide insightful and empathic feedback to one of the essays in this collection, as if you were the instructor.

8. Determine which of the reflections in this collection most appeals to you, and explain why.

9. Determine which of the reflections in this collection least appeals to you, and explain why.

Appendix II

Development of Student Professionalism

Mary T. Roth, Pharm.D., M.H.S.; and Thomas D. Zlatic, Ph.D.

In late 2007, the American College of Clinical Pharmacy (ACCP) charged their National StuNet Advisory Committee to formulate tenets of professionalism, with the primary goal of introducing students to essential attitudes and behaviors of professionalism. The committee's list of tenets served as a working document for the development of this White Paper. This collaborative effort of the ACCP Board of Regents and the National StuNet Advisory Committee sought to complement other published documents addressing student professionalism. The purpose of this White Paper is to enhance student understanding of professionalism, emphasizing the importance of the covenantal or "fiducial" relationship between the patient and the pharmacist. This fiducial relationship is the essence of professionalism and is a relationship between the patient and the pharmacist built on trust. This White Paper also outlines the traits of professionalism, which were developed after an extensive review of the literature on professionalism in medicine and pharmacy. The traits of professionalism identified here are responsibility, commitment to excellence, respect for others, honesty and integrity, and care and compassion. It is from these traits that student actions and behaviors should emanate. Students, pharmacy practitioners, and faculty have a responsibility to each other, to society as a whole, and to individual patients whom they serve to ensure that their words and actions uphold the highest standards of professional behavior.

Key Words: pharmacy students, professionalism, clinical pharmacy, American College of Clinical Pharmacy, ACCP.
(Pharmacotherapy 2009;29(6):749–756)

To assist students, pharmacy practitioners, and faculty in the development of student professionalism, the American College of Clinical Pharmacy (ACCP) charged their National StuNet Advisory Committee to formulate tenets of professionalism, with the primary goal of introducing students to the essential attitudes and behaviors of professionalism. The committee's list of tenets[1] served as a working document for the development of this White Paper. This collaborative effort of the ACCP Board of Regents and the National StuNet Advisory Committee seeks to complement other published documents addressing student professionalism.[2–5] The purpose of this White Paper is 3-fold:

- To enhance student understanding of professionalism, emphasizing the importance of the "fiducial" or covenantal relationship between the patient and pharmacist that lies at the heart of professionalism
- To introduce the traits of professionalism (Appendix 16–8) to students, explaining how these traits are linked to the fiducial relationship between the patient and pharmacist; it is from these traits that student actions and behaviors should emanate
- To stimulate discussion among students, pharmacy practitioners, and faculty as a means of fostering the development of student professionalism

The Essence of Professionalism

> *No physician, in so far as he is a physician, considers his own good in what he prescribes, but the good of his patient; for the true physician is also a ruler having the human body as a subject, and is not a mere money-maker.*
>
> Plato, *The Republic, Book I*

The profession of pharmacy is continually evolving to improve patient care. To uphold the ideals of the profession—to successfully care for and about patients—students must not only acquire the core clinical knowledge and skills, but also possess the attributes of a health care professional, namely, the attitudes, values, and habits that form the foundation of a profession. To accomplish this, they must first understand the uniqueness of a profession.

All definitions of "profession" are context sensitive and thus provisional; no single definition can encompass all applications. For instance, a baseball player or a dry cleaner may appropriately be labeled a professional, but these appellations do not convey the sense invoked here. In the traditional professions (medicine, law, education, and religion), the common features used to identify professions often include esoteric knowledge, self-regulation, a code of ethics, autonomy, and a service orientation.[9]

These features are elements within the definition of professionalism used here, but they do not in themselves distinguish a profession from an occupation. That essential difference was hinted at a decade ago when one author, searching for the "soul of pharmacy," provocatively asked whether pharmacy was an occupation or a profession.[10] His own response was that the evolution of pharmacy from occupational to professional status was dependent on the problematic transition from the product-oriented ethos of an occupation to the patient-oriented ethos of a profession.

In short, what essentially distinguishes a profession from an occupation is the relationship between the provider and the people being served.[9] In an occupation, the provider interacts with customers. In a profession, the professional provides care for patients, clients, congregations, or students. The difference between a customer and a client or patient is crucial. In an occupation, the relationship to a customer is commercial; the provider's first responsibility, appropriately, is to an employer or group of stockholders, although obviously, good business practice requires a balance between "caveat emptor" and "the customer is always right." Regardless, profit ultimately trumps all decisions. In a profession, the relationship between a provider and a recipient is not commercial but covenantal or fiducial. "Fiducial," derived from Latin word "fides," or faith, clearly affirms that faith and trust underlie professional interactions—a faith and trust that transcend occupational norms. In a profession, the provider has the knowledge and skills crucial to the well-being and even the life of the person seeking assistance. This person does not fully understand the knowledge base involved and cannot evaluate whether the services provided are the most effective. Thus, this individual must entrust the professional with his or her care and well-being: must give the "gift of trust." In return, the professional promises, by the very nature of the professional role, to act in the best interest of the patient.[11] This is the fiduciary or faith bond that undergirds professional services. If that bond is broken, the system fails.

The respect that the nonprofessional has for the professional is not based on the amount of money the professional makes or on social status, nor is it based on the amount of knowledge or quality of judgment he or she exhibits. Rather, the layperson respects the professional because he or she believes, and must believe, that the professional can be trusted to strive for the patient's well-being. Patients look to pharmacists as individuals who possess an in-depth knowledge of drugs. Patients trust that pharmacists will provide personalized, up-to-date, clinically relevant, and useful information about their drugs to improve their health and prevent them harm. The patient's trust in the pharmacist as a professional and the pharmacist's acting in the best interest of the patient at all times bind this relationship and define pharmacy as a true profession.

Traits of Professionalism
Working from the concept of a "profession" that is based on a patient-centered ethos—that is, on fiducial or covenantal responsibilities—we can begin detailing the essential traits of a professional.

In our review of the literature, we identified several related constructs and characteristics that could have easily been listed among the cognitive, emotive, attitudinal, ethical, and behavioral traits of professionals, including empathy, reliability, collaboration, cooperation, advocacy, professional competence, altruism, creativity, innovation, and leadership (to name a few).[2-5, 9-14] Although all of these characteristics are desirable goals for a student professional, instructors' remarks to students to "act professionally" are often simply admonitions to improve civility, demeanor, language, and physical appearance: "Be quiet, please"; "Come to class on time"; "Avoid slang"; "Enunciate more clearly"; "Wear clothing that is more appropriate." Moreover, although such breaches of professionalism are, of course, not trivial, students should gain the ability to discern the underlying principles and reasons for such behaviors. Hence, our purpose is to identify a manageable core of essential traits that form a substructure for instilling student professionalism. At stake is the public trust, which is essential for providing quality patient care.

The traits of professionalism in Appendix I were developed after an extensive review of the literature on professionalism in medicine, nursing, and pharmacy.[2-5, 11-15] In addition, our articulation of the traits relied on input from the ACCP National StuNet Advisory Committee, as well as review and critique by several professionals and the ACCP Board of Regents.[1] Of note, most of the characteristics, tenets, or qualities of professionalism identified in the literature are connected to the fiducial relationship between the patient and pharmacist, and all are important. Our goal in compiling the traits of professionalism was to be comprehensive, yet to arrive at the traits that might best capture the essence of professionalism without losing sight of the important contribution of related characteristics.

To illustrate and explain the relationship between the traits of professionalism and the patient-pharmacist fiducial relationship, we expand on an analogy suggested by a previously published article entitled "Student Professionalism."[4] As a simple way to conceptualize professionalism, envision a bicycle wheel (Figure 1). We propose that

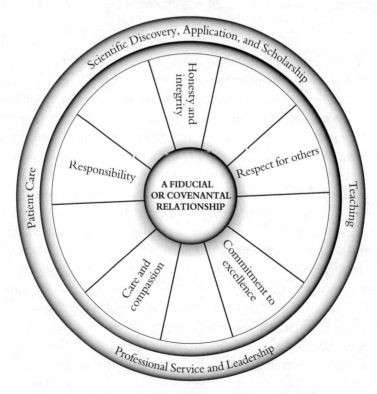

Figure 1. Conceptualizing professionalism in pharmacy.

the hub of the wheel is the heart of professionalism, the fiducial or covenantal relationship that pharmacists have with the patients whom they serve. The spokes of the wheel are the traits of professionalism, from which professional behaviors and actions should emanate. Traits of professionalism include assuming responsibility, demonstrating a commitment to excellence, respecting others, displaying honesty and integrity, and demonstrating care and compassion. The tire is literally "where the rubber meets the road"—a road that leads to patient care; teaching; scientific discovery, application, and scholarship; and professional service and leadership. Although the physical appearance and image of the bicycle are important and should not be overlooked (i.e., how professionals dress, carry themselves, and represent themselves in interactions with others), the essential part of professionalism is the hub of the wheel put into action by the spokes—without a relationship built on trust and the actions and behaviors exemplifying this trust, the tire itself and the road traveled are no longer those of a professional.

Exercising Professionalism
What one says and does, how one treats others, and how one conducts oneself on a daily basis convey character. Students must be committed to the development of professionalism, thereby assuming responsibility for exercising the appropriate professional behaviors throughout their pharmacy education and training. Similarly, as members of society, pharmacists must remember that they are professionals, trusted by the students they teach, the colleagues with whom they interact, the community and public at-large who depend on their expertise, and, most important, the patients they serve. Pharmacists must be committed to upholding the highest standards of professional behavior.

Students may pursue a wide range of professional opportunities after graduation from pharmacy school. Many will provide direct patient care and experience firsthand the importance of maintaining the highest standards of professional behavior in daily interactions with patients. Emphasis should be placed on the critical role of professionalism in the provision of patient care: the trusting relationship and covenantal bond between pharmacist and patient that defines pharmacy as a profession. In the words of one author, it is the pharmacy practitioners who have internalized the core values of the profession and who have made personal commitments to establishing these relationships and moving the profession forward.[16] On entry into the profession, students may also pursue opportunities not involving direct patient care, as entrepreneurs, pharmacy managers, pharmacists working in various capacities within industry and government, administrators in hospitals and other organizations, and scientists devoting their careers to improving drug therapy outcomes. Even though, in these capacities, individual pharmacist-patient relationships are not the focus, these professional roles ultimately improve the lives of patients. Despite their separation from direct patient care, these pharmacists also must internalize the core values of the profession and make personal commitments to moving the profession forward; in brief, it is essential that they, too, exhibit the traits of professionalism that define pharmacy as a true profession.

Teaching Professionalism

The crucial question, then, is what in pharmacy education prepares students for such responsibilities—what informs and motivates students to achieve a professional identity? Teaching and assessing professionalism within a curriculum is a Herculean challenge. For more than 3 decades, new methods have been introduced for engaging students and promoting active learning in the classroom. These methods include interactive learning environments with standardized patients, which provide opportunities for students to practice and refine their skills, and innovative clinical training settings that expose students to real-world clinical care for patients of all ages. In pharmacy,[17–22] as well as across medical professions,[13–15, 23–32] numerous strategies have been developed to enhance curricular efforts aimed at promoting professionalism.

Yet, even though curricular efforts to enhance professionalism may be effective, they are not sufficient. Pedagogy has long known that in education, there is a "hidden curriculum," a process of socialization that enculturates students, instilling values, habits, attitudes, paradigms, and biases—much of it transmitted unknowingly using no formal systems. In pharmacy, as in medicine, "although matters of technical information and the transmission of technical skills traditionally have been thought to lie at the heart of the medical educational system, medical training at root is a process of moral enculturation; in transmitting normative rules regarding behavior and emotions to its trainees, the medical school functions as a moral community."[32]

This hidden curriculum of unwritten and unspoken guidelines for belief and behavior can be a tremendous tool for furthering professional development. Exposure to the role modeling of professionalism throughout one's pharmacy education and training is probably more effective than weeks of lectures. It is through modeling—the student's exposure to what pharmacy practitioners and faculty actually say and do in day-to-day interactions with one another and with patients—that professional development occurs. Such role modeling serves as the most powerful influence on a student's understanding of professionalism.[14]

Another, more subtle opportunity for role modeling presents itself in the classroom or experiential site. A teacher, like a pharmacist, is a professional. The teacher-as-professional is obligated to support a fiducial relationship with students.[9] The teacher's primary obligation is to the student—to help the student succeed in his or her learning. Entailed in that fiducial relationship are respect, care, and empathy for the student. If students sense that the instructor is committed to and concerned about their welfare, they can experience firsthand, and appreciate, what a fiducial commitment means.

However, instructors who exhibit arrogance, indifference, or aloofness to patients or students also educate and enlighten students about professional roles. Wise students perhaps can learn from these negative examples and thus progress in professional development (students can learn professionalism by observing its breach), but for others, the negative behaviors become ensconced in their understanding of professional roles. They learn from the modeling, but what they learn is different from what they are lectured on in the classroom. Thus, unfortunately, there is a downside to the hidden curriculum. If unexamined and uncontrolled, it can interfere with the student's development of the traits defining professionalism that are requisite for patient care.

Throughout one's pharmacy education and training, professionalism should be discussed, evaluated, and, most important, modeled. In their daily interactions with students, faculty must demonstrate the traits of professionalism: responsibility, commitment to excellence, respect for others, honesty and integrity, and care and compassion. Faculty must hold students accountable for their behaviors and actions and guide them toward developing their own excellence in professionalism. Students must recognize poor examples of faculty and pharmacist modeling (i.e., what not to do and how not to act) and commit to providing a better example. Similarly, students should recognize and internalize exemplars of true professionalism and, in turn, instill these values in others. Students have a responsibility to ensure that their words and actions in the classroom, at the bedside, and before society as a whole uphold the highest standards of professional behavior. Faculty and practitioners must do the same.

Conclusion

It is important that students, pharmacy practitioners, and faculty recognize what is truly at the heart of professionalism—the pharmacist-patient fiducial or covenantal relationship. Professionalism is driven by much more than one's actions and behaviors—professionalism hinges on a trust relationship. The pharmacist-patient fiducial or covenantal relationship obligates the pharmacist to act in the best interest of the patient. As a result, the patient has a firm belief, an unwavering trust that the pharmacist will provide him or her with the best possible care. The traits of professionalism (responsibility, commitment to excellence, respect for others, honesty and integrity, care and compassion) should be discussed, practiced, and, most important, modeled. Students, pharmacy practitioners, and faculty have a responsibility to each other, to society as a whole, and to the individual patients and students whom they serve to ensure that their words and actions both within and outside the classroom uphold the highest standards of professional behavior.

References

1. American College of Clinical Pharmacy. Tenets of professionalism for pharmacy students. Pharmacotherapy 2009 (6);29:757–759.
2. Hammer DP. Professional attitudes and behaviors: the "A's and B's" of professionalism. Am J Pharm Educ 2000;64:455–64.
3. American Pharmaceutical Association Academy of Students of Pharmacy—American Association of Colleges of Pharmacy Council of Deans Task Force on Professionalism. White paper on pharmacy student professionalism. J Am Pharm Assoc 2000;40:96–102.

4. Hammer DP, Berger BA, Beardsley RS, Easton MR. Student professionalism. Am J Pharm Educ 2003;67:1–29.
5. American Society of Health-System Pharmacists. ASHP statement on professionalism. Am J Health Syst Pharm 2008;65:172–4.
6. Sharpe VA. Behind closed doors: accountability and responsibility in patient care. J Med Philos 2000;25:28–47.
7. Leininger M. Leininger's theory of nursing: cultural care diversity and universality. Nurs Sci Q 1988;1:152–60.
8. Galt KA. The need to define care in pharmaceutical care: an examination across research, practice and education. Am J Pharm Educ 2000;64:223–33.
9. Zlatic TD, ed. The professional nature of teaching. In: Re-visioning professional education: an orientation to teaching. Kansas City, MO: American College of Clinical Pharmacy, 2005:5–10.
10. Zellmer WA. Searching for the soul of pharmacy. Am J Health Syst Pharm 1996;53:1911–16.
11. American Pharmacists Association. Code of ethics for pharmacists. Available from http://www.pharmacist.com/AM/Template.cfm?Section=Code_of_Ethics_for_Pharmacists&Template=/CM/HTMLDisplay.cfm&ContentID=5420. Accessed December 16, 2008.
12. American Association of Colleges of Pharmacy. Oath of a pharmacist. Available from http://www.aacp.org/Docs/Main Navigation/ForDeans/9517_OATHOFAPHARMACIST2008–09.pdf. Accessed December 16, 2008.
13. American Board of Internal Medicine. Project professionalism, 2001. Available from http://www.abim.org/pdf/publications/ professionalism.pdf. Accessed December 16, 2008.
14. Inui T. A flag in the wind: educating for professionalism in medicine. Washington, DC: Association of American Medical Colleges, 2003. Available from www.regenstrief.org/bio/ professionalism.pdf/download. Accessed December 16, 2008.
15. Brainard AH, Brislen HC. Learning professionalism: a view from the trenches. Acad Med 2007;82:1010–14.
16. Zellmer WA, ed. Pharmacy's professional imperative: distinguishing between pharmacy providers and practitioners. In: The conscience of a pharmacist: essays on vision and leadership for a profession. Bethesda, MD: American Society of Health-System Pharmacists, Inc., 2002:1–3.
17. Chisholm MA, Cobb H, Duke L, McDuffie C, Kennedy WK. Development of an instrument to measure professionalism. Am J Pharm Educ 2006;70:1–6.
18. Bumgarner GW, Spies AR, Asbill CS, Prince VT. Using the humanities to strengthen the concept of professionalism among first-professional year pharmacy students. Am J Pharm Educ 2007;71:1–6.
19. Duncan-Hewitt W. The development of a professional: reinterpretation of the professionalization problem from the perspective of cognitive/moral development. Am J Pharm Educ 2005;69:44–54.
20. Purkerson Hammer D, Mason HL, Chalmers RK, Popovich NG, Rupp MT. Development and testing of an instrument to assess behavioral professionalism of pharmacy students. Am J Pharm Educ 2000;64:141–51.
21. Brehm B, Breen P, Brown B, et al. Instructional design and assessment: an interdisciplinary approach to introducing professionalism. Am J Pharm Educ 2006;70:1–5.
22. Sylvia LM. Enhancing professionalism of pharmacy students: results of a national survey. Am J Pharm Educ 2004;68:1–12.
23. Adams D, Miller B. Professionalism in nursing behaviors of nurse practitioners. J Prof Nurs 2001;17:203–10.

24. American Physical Therapy Association. Professionalism in physical therapy: core values self-assessment. Alexandria, VA: American Physical Therapy Association, 2003. Available from http://www.apta.org/AM/Template.cfm?Section=Home&CONTENTID=41461&TEMPLATE=/CM/ContentDisplay.cfm. Accessed December 16, 2008.

25. Cornett BS. A principal calling: professionalism and health care services. J Commun Disord 2006;39:301–9.

26. Wear D, Bickel J, eds. Educating for professionalism: creating a culture of humanism in medical education. Ames, IA: University of Iowa Press, 2000.

27. Epstein RM, Hundert EM. Defining and assessing professional competence. JAMA 2002;287:226–35.

28. Hatern C. Teaching approaches that reflect and promote professionalism. Acad Med 2003;78:709–13.

29. Hickson GB, Pichert JW, Webb LE, Gabbe SG. A complementary approach to promoting professionalism: identifying, measuring, and addressing unprofessional behaviors. Acad Med 2007;82:1040–8.

30. Lynch D, Surdyk P, Eiser A. Assessing professionalism: a review of the literature. Med Teach 2004;26:366–73.

31. Rees CE, Knight LV. The trouble with assessing students' professionalism: theoretical insights from sociocognitive psychology. Acad Med 2007;82:46–50.

32. Hafferty FW, Franks R. The hidden curriculum, ethics teaching, and the structure of medical education. Acad Med 1994;69:861–71.

Contributors

Maurice D. Alexander, Pharm.D.
University of North Carolina Hospitals and Clinics
North Carolina Cancer Hospital

Shari Allen, Pharm.D.
Assistant Professor of Pharmacy Practice
Philadelphia College of Osteopathic
Medicine—School of Pharmacy

Sally A. Arif, Pharm.D., BCPS
Assistant Professor of Pharmacy Practice
Midwestern University
Chicago College of Pharmacy

Richard J. Artymowicz,
Pharm.D., FCCP, BCPS
Cape Regional Medical Center

Jennifer M. Belavic, Pharm.D., FASCP
University of Pittsburgh Medical
Center—Presbyterian Hospital

Jeffrey M. Brewer, Pharm.D.
Associate Professor, Family Medicine
Department of Pharmacy Practice
Albany College of Pharmacy and Health Sciences

Kyle Burghardt, Pharm.D.
Department of Clinical, Social and
Administrative Services
University of Michigan College of Pharmacy

Brooke D. Butler, Pharm.D.
PGY1 Pharmacy Practice Resident
Carl Vinson VA Medical Center

Louis L. Bystrak, Pharm.D., BCPS, BCOP
Clinical/Staff Pharmacist
Women & Children's Hospital of
Buffalo/Kaleida Health
Adjunct Instructor, Department of Pharmacy
The University at Buffalo School of Pharmacy
and Pharmaceutical Sciences

Amanda C. Chuk, Pharm.D., BCPS
Clinical Pharmacist Specialist – Critical Care
Dartmouth-Hitchcock Medical Center

Valerie Azzopardi Coppenrath,
Pharm.D., BCPS
Assistant Professor of Pharmacy Practice
Massachusetts College of Pharmacy
and Health Sciences
School of Pharmacy—Worcester/Manchester

Lindsay Davison, Pharm.D.
Food and Drug Administration
Center for Drug Evaluation and Research
Office of Communications
Division of Drug Information

Paul Denvir, Ph.D.
Assistant Professor, Department
of Arts and Sciences
Albany College of Pharmacy and Health Sciences

Melissa Dinolfo, Pharm.D., BCOP
Director of Pharmacy and Clinic Operations
Premiere Oncology

Robert Draeger, Pharm.D.
James L. Winkle College of Pharmacy
University of Cincinnati

Ashley Wimberly Ellis, Pharm.D.
Clinical Assistant Professor of Pharmacy Practice
University of Mississippi School of Pharmacy

Erica Estus, Pharm D., CGP
Clinical Assistant Professor, Department
of Pharmacy Practice
University of Rhode Island School of Pharmacy

Katherine R. Fitz, Pharm.D.
Riverside Methodist Hospital, OhioHealth

Alex Flannery, Pharm.D.
University of Kentucky College of Pharmacy

Peter Gal, Pharm.D.
Director, Graduate Pharmacy Education
Greensboro Area Health Education Center
Director, Neonatal Pharmacotherapy Fellowship
Women's Hospital/Cone Health
Clinical Professor, DPPEE, Eshelman
School of Pharmacy
University of North Carolina at Chapel Hill

Shannon H. Goldwater,
  Pharm.D., FASHP, BCPS
Clinical Assistant Professor, School of Pharmacy
Virginia Commonwealth University
Preceptor, School of Pharmacy
Shenandoah University
Adjunct Assistant Professor, School of Pharmacy
Howard University

Seena L. Haines, Pharm.D., BC-
  ADM, FAPhA, FASHP, CDE
Professor and Associate Dean for Faculty
Gregory School of Pharmacy
Palm Beach Atlantic University

Nicole J. Harger, Pharm.D., BCPS
UC Health—University Hospital

Kristin Held, Pharm.D., BCOP
Children's Mercy Hospitals and Clinics

Joel Henneberry
Pharm.D. Candidate 2012
St. Louis College of Pharmacy

Amber Holdiness, Pharm.D.
Clinical Pharmacist
Bon Secours St. Francis Health System

Charnicia E. Huggins, Pharm.D., M.S.
University at Buffalo, The State
  University of New York

Stephen W. Janning, Pharm.D.
Director of Clinical Development
GlaxoSmithKline

Lauren J. Jonkman, Pharm.D., BCPS

Kelly Kabat, Pharm.D., BCPS

Kristi Kelley, Pharm.D., BCPS, CDE
Associate Clinical Professor of Pharmacy Practice
Auburn University Harrison School of Pharmacy
Clinical Pharmacist
Continuity Clinics with Baptist Health System

William Klugh Kennedy,
  Pharm.D., BCPP, FASHP
Pharmacy Practice and Behavioral Medicine
Mercer University/Memorial
  University Medical Center

Chad A. Knoderer, Pharm.D.
Butler University College of Pharmacy
  and Health Sciences

Marianne E. Koenig, Pharm.D., BCPS
Assistant Professor, Department of
  Pharmacotherapeutics and Clinical Research
Coordinator of Clinical Academic Simulation
University of South Florida College of Pharmacy

Judith L. Kristeller, Pharm.D., BCPS
Associate Professor, Department
  of Pharmacy Practice
Wilkes University

Bonnie A. Labdi, Pharm.D., R.Ph.
Baptist Hospitals of Southeast Texas

Virginia A. Lemay, Pharm.D., CDOE
University of Rhode Island College of Pharmacy

Adrienne J. Lindblad, Pharm.D.,
  BSP, BSc, ACPR
Clinical Practice Leader
Alberta Health Services

J. Christopher Lynch, Pharm.D.
Professor of Pharmacy Practice
Edwardsville School of Pharmacy
Southern Illinois University

Karen F. Marlowe, Pharm.D., BCPS, CPE
Auburn University Harrison School of Pharmacy
University of South Alabama School of Medicine

Katie S. McClendon, Pharm.D., BCPS
Clinical Assistant Professor
University of Mississippi School of Pharmacy

Jane McLaughlin-Middlekauff, Pharm.D.
Assistant Professor, Pharmacy Practice
Nova Southeastern University

Gary Milavetz, Pharm.D., B.S.
Associate Professor, Division of Pharmaceutics
  and Translational Therapeutics
Department of Pharmaceutical Sciences
  and Experimental Therapeutics
College of Pharmacy, The University of Iowa

Deborah S. Minor, Pharm.D.
Professor
University of Mississippi Medical Center
School of Medicine

Candis M. Morello, Pharm.D., CDE
Associate Professor of Clinical Pharmacy
Associate Dean for Student Affairs
UC San Diego, Skaggs School of Pharmacy
  and Pharmaceutical Sciences
Clinical Pharmacist Specialist
Veterans Affairs San Diego Healthcare System

Benyam Muluneh, Pharm.D.
University of North Carolina Hospitals and Clinics
North Carolina Cancer Hospital

John E. Murphy, Pharm.D., BSPharm
Professor and Associate Dean,
  Pharmacy Practice and Science
The University of Arizona College of Pharmacy

Ricky Ogden, Pharm.D., BCPS
Children's Mercy Hospitals and Clinics

Margie Padilla, Pharm.D., CDE
University of Texas at El Paso
UTEP/UT Austin Cooperative Pharmacy Program

Adam Pate, Pharm.D.
Clinical Assistant Professor
University of Louisiana at Monroe
  College of Pharmacy

Kristen Pate, Pharm.D.
Clinical Assistant Professor
University of Louisiana at Monroe
  College of Pharmacy

Kimberly A. Pesaturo, Pharm.D., BCPS
Assistant Professor of Pharmacy Practice
School of Pharmacy—Worcester/Manchester
Massachusetts College of Pharmacy
  and Health Sciences

Doreen Pon, Pharm.D., BCOP
Assistant Professor of Pharmacy
  Practice and Administration
Western University of Health Sciences,
  College of Pharmacy
Faculty in Residence
City of Hope National Medical Center

Charles D. Ponte, Pharm.D, BSc,
  DPNAP, FAPhA, FASHP, FCCP
Robert C. Byrd Health Sciences Center
Schools of Pharmacy and Medicine
West Virginia University

Anna Miszczanczuk Portakalis, Pharm.D.

Lisa Powell, Pharm.D.
Pharmacy Department
Moses Cone Memorial Hospital

Brandi Puet, Pharm.D.
Aegis Sciences Corporation

Laurie L. Pylitt, M.H.P.E., PA-C
Associate Professor, Director of Assessment
Butler University College of Pharmacy
  and Health Sciences

Frances M. Rodríguez, Pharm.D., BCPS
Associate Professor and Chair,
  Pharmacy Practice Department
School of Pharmacy
University of Puerto Rico

Karl Ruch, Pharm.D., BCPS
Pharmacist, NICU/Peds Service Line
Mission Hospitals

Kayce M. Shealy, Pharm.D., BCPS
Presbyterian College School of Pharmacy

Keri A. Sims, Pharm.D., BCPS

Brenda T. Smith, R.Ph., PIC, M.S.
Director of Experiential Education
  and Assistant Professor
Appalachian College of Pharmacy
Pharmacist-in-Charge, Mountain Care Center

Kayla E. Smith, Pharm.D.

Roger W. Sommi, Pharm.D., FCCP, BCPP
Professor of Pharmacy Practice and Psychiatry
Schools of Pharmacy and Medicine
University of Missouri—Kansas City

Brandon Sucher, Pharm.D., CDE, AE-C
Associate Professor of Pharmacy Practice
Regis University School of Pharmacy

Courtney L. Tam, Pharm.D.
Health-System Pharmacy Administration
Richard L. Roudebush VA Medical Center

Rebecca A. Taylor, Pharm.D., MBA, BCPS
Cleveland Clinic Education Manager
Assistant Professor, Department
  of Pharmacy Practice
Northeast Ohio Medical University

Betty Ann Torres, Pharm.D.
Associate Professor, Pharmacy
  Practice Department
School of Pharmacy
University of Puerto Rico

Joy Vongspanich, Pharm.D.
UC Davis Medical Center

Ann McMahon Wicker, Pharm.D., BCPS

Jon P. Wietholter, Pharm.D., BCPS
Clinical Assistant Professor
West Virginia University

Lori Wilken, Pharm.D., B.S.
University of Illinois at Chicago

Felix K. Yam, Pharm.D.
Clinical Assistant Professor, Health Sciences
UC San Diego Skaggs School of Pharmacy
  and Pharmaceutical Sciences

Christine K. Yocum, Pharm.D.

Donald Zabriskie, BPharm, MBA, RPh
Cleveland Clinic—Fairview Hospital

William A. Zellmer, B.S.
  (Pharmacy), M.P.H.
President, Pharmacy Foresight

Thomas D. Zlatic, Ph.D.
Professor, Department of Liberal Arts
  and Administrative Sciences
St. Louis College of Pharmacy